Addictive Prescription Drugs

Find Out What's Hiding in the Fine Print

Vital information for
Every Patient, Friend and Caregiver

Compiled and
Written in Plain English by
Meridith Berk

Table of Contents

Introduction

Many people think because a drug is legal and prescribed by a doctor the drug must be good for you and cannot be addictive or dangerous. Unfortunately this isn't true. Many prescription drugs especially, painkillers, sedatives and stimulants can be highly addictive. Part of what makes an addictive drug so difficult to come off of is the powerful and often painful withdrawal symptoms that accompany any attempt to quit.

With mood and behavior drugs this can make it seem like you need to take them or that you'll get sick without them. Many times this feeling is simply the result of withdrawals. Withdrawing from any drug can easily make you feel you were better off taking it. Look at the number of people who cannot quit smoking even though it has been proven time after time that smoking kills. Yet when someone is addicted to smoking (which most smokers are) they do anything possible to ignore the dangers because they don't want to go through the intense mental and physical discomfort of withdrawal.

The bottom line is that a legally prescribed drug is not necessarily safe or non-addictive. This is why it is of such importance that anyone being prescribed a drug find out for themselves the side effects and warnings attached to that medication, as well as how likely it is for them to become addicted to it.

Many prescription drugs are just as addictive as or more addictive than any street drug. Care should be taken with these drugs both in starting them and in withdrawing from them. It should be noted that due to their level of addictiveness you should take into account both the potential side effects and the potential withdrawal symptoms before filling that prescription and always ask your doctor if any other approach or treatment can be tried first before starting any drug. If your doctor doesn't know, get a second opinion. It's *your* health that's at stake.

According to the FDA, many drugs don't cure the condition for which they're prescribed. They treat the condition or possibly lessen the symptoms. It's important to make sure you understand if the medication you are about to start taking will cure the condition that is bothering you or will just possible lessen symptoms. This, as well as whether it can be addictive, may have a bearing on whether you want to start taking the drug or would rather find out if there is an alternative treatment for your condition.

Find out all you can about the medication and always ask yourself if the benefit is worth the risk.

Included in this booklet are both prescription drugs which are stated as being habit-forming by the FDA and those drugs, while they may not actually be addictive, need to be withdrawn from gradually and under medical supervision.

With the thousands of drugs that have been approved by the FDA I cannot say these are all the addictive prescription drugs. I have tried to include the most used of these drugs.

If you do not see a drug you are taking or are about to take listed in this booklet DO NOT assume that you can quit taking it without potential problems or that it's not addictive.

Talk to your doctor or qualified health professional before you stop taking any prescription drug.

In order to give some additional cautionary information I have included a section on special warnings connected with many of the drugs. The actual side effects, overdose symptoms, warnings, reasons for not prescribing and cautions to prescribers are listed on the label connected to the drug and can also be found at the U.S. Government's MedlinePlus web site found at: www.nlm.nih.gov/medlineplus/medlineplus.html

With prescription drug addiction at an all time high in the United States and deaths from both legal and illegal drugs on the rise it's a good time to think twice before leaving your doctor's office with a prescription. Ask your doctor for additional options. If you get no help, ask another physician until you find one who is willing to work with you in finding the simplest and least dangerous solution that works for you.

Please note that this booklet in no way takes the place of seeing a qualified medical professional. It also does not contain nearly all the information available on these drugs. Don't make decisions based solely on the information provided here. Talk to a doctor.

Drugs are listed first in alphabetical order by brand name, the alphabetically by generic or chemical name.

Addictive Pharmaceutical Drugs

Alphabetically by Brand Name

Brand Name: Actiq
Generic Name: fentanyl

Type or Class of Drug: Opiate (narcotic) pain reliever
A narcotic is a substance that dulls pain and induces sleep. Opiate means that is derived from or acts like opium in dulling the senses and inducing sleep.

Approved for: Breakthrough pain from cancer. Breakthrough pain is sudden episodes of pain that occur despite round the clock treatment with pain medication.

Dependency and Addiction: This drug may become habit-forming, however since Actiq is used for the treatment of chronic cancer pain the National Library of Medicine DailyMed web site recommends that fear of tolerance and physical dependence should not deter using high enough doses to adequately relieve the pain. According to this same web site physical dependence is not ordinarily a concern when one is treating a patient with chronic cancer pain.

Do not stop taking Actiq without talking to your doctor. The physical dependence associated with this drug results in withdrawal symptoms in patients who abruptly stop taking Actiq.

Withdrawals:

Symptoms of withdrawal include:

Abdominal cramping
Agitation (suddenly violent and forceful, emotionally disturbed state of mind)
Anxiety
Diarrhea
Dilated pupils
Goose bumps

Increased tearing
Insomnia
Muscle aches
Nausea
Runny nose
Sweating
Vomiting
Yawning

Important Warnings: The Black Box Warning (Special FDA Warning) for Actiq includes but is not limited to the following:

Actiq contains a medicine in an amount which can be fatal to a child. Death has been reported in children who have accidentally ingested Actiq.

Actiq is intended to be used only in the care of cancer patients and only by oncologists and pain specialists who are knowledgeable of and skilled in the use of opioids to treat cancer pain. (An opioid is a drug with similar properties to opium. Opioids are drugs used for pain management.)

Opioid painkillers now cause more drug overdose deaths than cocaine and heroin combined.

Information on side effects, overdose symptoms and other special warnings can be found by visiting either of the National Library of Medicine web sites listed in the reference section at the end of this booklet.

Brand Name: Adderall / Adderall XR
Generic Name: amphetamine / dextroamphetamine

Type or Class of Drug: Central Nervous System Stimulant

[A stimulant is a drug that increases heart rate, breathing rate, brain function. And nervous system.]

Approved for: Treatment of ADHD in adults and children and for treatment of narcolepsy (asleep disorder that causes excessive sleepiness during the daytime and sudden attacks of sleep)

Dependency and Addiction: Adderall and Adderall XR can be habit-forming. Amphetamines (one of the ingredients in Adderall) have a high potential for abuse. Taking amphetamines for a prolonged period may lead to drug dependence. The drugs should be prescribed and dispensed sparingly.

Amphetamines have been extensively abused. Tolerance, extreme dependence and severe social disability have occurred.

Withdrawals:

Abruptly stopping this drug after taking high doses can result in withdrawal symptoms including:

Severe dermatoses (Skin problems)
Depression
Extreme fatigue
Hyperactivity (a condition characterized by excessive restlessness and movement)
Insomnia
Irritability
Personality changes
Psychosis, often indistinguishable from schizophrenia (psychosis is defined as a loss of contact with reality where the person gets false ideas about what is taking place or who he is and has hallucinations, seeing or hearing things that aren'there)

Important Warnings: Adderall and Adderall XR have many warnings including the FDA's Black Box Warning. These warnings include:

Misuse of amphetamines may cause sudden death and serious cardiovascular adverse events (like heart attacks).

Dextroamphetamine and amphetamine may slow children's growth or weight gain.

If you take too much dextroamphetamine and amphetamine, you may find that the medication no longer controls your symptoms

You may feel a need to take large amounts of the medication.

You may experience symptoms such as rash, difficulty falling asleep or staying asleep, irritability, hyperactivity, and unusual changes in your personality or behavior.

Overusing Adderall or Adderall XR may also cause sudden death or serious heart problems such as heart attack or stroke.

Even if you or your child or loved one is taking exactly the amount prescribed, please be aware of the above important warnings and contact your doctor immediately if any of the above should occur.

Remember this drug is addictive and included in the effects of taking too much are changes in the patient's personality or behavior. So extra caution should be taken to contact a doctor the moment you sense any possible change.

Since this drug is often abused it's important to keep track of how many tablets or capsules are left so you will know if any are missing.

This medication also may cause sudden death, heart attack, or stroke in adults, especially adults with heart defects or serious heart problems.

Adderall and Adderall XR may cause sudden death in children and teenagers, especially children and teenagers who have heart defects or serious heart problems.

Brand Name: Ambien
Generic Name: zolpidem

Type or Class: Sedative - hypnotic

Approved for: Treatment of insomnia

Dependency and Addiction: "If you take zolpidem for 2 weeks or longer, zolpidem may not help you sleep as well as it did when you first began to take the medication. If you take zolpidem for a long time, you also may develop dependence ('addiction,' a need to continue taking the medication) on zolpidem." From MedlinePlus web site

Signs of addiction include impaired control over drug use, compulsive drug use, continued use despite harm and craving.

Withdrawals: If you suddenly stop taking zolpidem, you may develop unpleasant feelings or you may experience more severe withdrawal symptoms such as:

Abdominal cramps
Convulsions (Uncontrolled shaking of the body, a seizure)
Dysphoria (a state of anxiety, depression, unease)
Fatigue
Flushing
Insomnia
Lightheadedness
Muscle cramps
Nausea
Nervousness
Panic attacks
Seizures
Shakiness
Stomach
Sweating
Tremors
Uncontrolled crying
Vomiting

Important Warnings:

Ambien (zolpidem) may make you drowsy during the day and may increase the risk that you could fall.

Take care not to drive a car or operate machinery until you know how Ambien affects you.

Alcohol can make the side affects from Ambien worse.

Some people who took zolpidem got out of bed and drove their cars, prepared and ate food, had sex, made phone calls, or were involved in other activities while partially asleep. After they woke up, these people were usually unable to remember what they had done. Call your doctor right away if you find out that you have been driving or doing anything else unusual while you were sleeping.

Your mental health may change in unexpected ways while you are taking this medication. Notify your doctor right away if experience any of the following serious symptoms. :

Aggressiveness
Confusion
Difficulty concentrating
Extroversion that seems out of character
Hallucinations (seeing things or hearing voices that do not exist)
Feeling as if you are outside of your body
Memory problems
New or worsening depression
Slowed speech or movements
Strange or unusually outgoing behavior
Suicidal behavior
Thinking about killing yourself
Any other changes in your usual thoughts
Any other changes in your usual mood
Any other changes in your usual behavior

Be sure that your family knows these symptoms so that they can call the doctor if you are unable to seek treatment on your own.

Safety and effectiveness of Ambien have not been established in children. Many children (7.4%) given Ambien in clinical trials hallucinated (saw or heard things that were not there).

Brand Name: Ativan
Generic Name: lorazepam

Type or Class of Drug: Benzodiazepine - Minor Sedative
(One of the types of drugs used as tranquilizers or sedatives or hypnotics or muscle relaxants; chronic use can lead to dependency)

Approved for: Relieving anxiety. It's also used to treat irritable bowel syndrome, epilepsy, insomnia, and nausea and vomiting from cancer treatment and to control agitation caused by alcohol withdrawal.

Dependency and Addiction: Lorazepam can be habit-forming. Do not take a larger dose, take it more often, or for a longer time than your doctor tells you to. Tolerance may develop with long-term or excessive use, making the drug less effective. Do not take lorazepam for more than 4 months or stop taking this medication without talking to your doctor.

Withdrawals:

Do not suddenly stop taking this drug. Stopping the drug suddenly can worsen your condition. You will need to come off this drug gradually in order to control the withdrawal symptoms which include:

Abdominal cramps
Agitation (suddenly violent and forceful, emotionally disturbed state of mind)
Anxiety
Anxiousness
Confusion
Convulsions

Delirium (a temporary state of extreme mental confusion which can include anxiety, disorientation, hallucinations, delusions, and incoherent speech.

Depression

Depersonalization (feeling of no longer being an individual or no longer being yourself - feeling of watching oneself act and having no control over what one is doing)

Derealization (condition where the external world seems strange or unreal)

Diarrhea
Dizziness
Dysphoria (a state of anxiety, depression ,unease)
Hallucinations
Headache
Hyperacusis (Impaired ability to tolerate normal environmental sounds)
Hyperreflexia (overactive or over-responsive reflexes. Examples can include twitching or spastic tendencies)
Hypersensitivity to light (hyper means exaggerated or too much, extreme, above normal)
Hypersensitivity to noise (hyper means exaggerated or too much, extreme, above normal)
Hypersensitivity to perceptual changes (hyper means exaggerated or too much, extreme, above normal)
Hypersensitivity to physical contact (hyper means exaggerated or too much, extreme, above normal)
Hyperthermia (abnormally high body temperature usually the result of head injury, medication or infection)
Insomnia
Involuntary movements
Irritability
Loss of appetite
Myalgia (muscle pain)
Nausea
Numbness of extremities

Palpitations (heartbeat sensations that feel like your heart is pounding or racing)

Panic attacks

Rebound phenomena (the tendency of a medication, when discontinued, to cause a return of the symptoms being treated to be more severe than before)

Restlessness
Seizures
Short term memory loss
Sleeplessness
Sweating
Tachycardia (a rapid heart rate)
Tension
Tingling of extremities
Tremors
Vertigo
Vomiting

Some symptoms of Ativan withdrawal have not been listed on the government web sites used as primary research for this booklet. More symptoms of Ativan withdrawal can be found at: www.prozactruth.com/ativan.htm

Do not suddenly stop taking Ativan. Your doctor probably will decrease your dose gradually.

Important Warnings:

In patients who are depressed a possibility for suicide should be borne in mind.

Lorazepam should be used with caution in patients with any sort of respiratory (breathing) or lung problems.

Special caution, elderly or debilitated patients may be more susceptible to the sedative effects of Ativan (lorazepam). Sedative means the reduction of anxiety, stress, irritability, or excitement.

Paradoxical reactions have occasionally been reported during use. These reactions are more likely to occur in children and the elderly. Should this occur, use of the drug should be stopped. A paradoxical reaction is when the drug produces the opposite effect as is expected. So if a person has a paradoxical reaction to a drug that is supposed to have a calming effect the drug will instead produce anxiety.

Brand Name: Buspar
Generic Name: buspirone

Type or Class of Drug: Anti-anxiety

Approved for: Short-term treatment for relief of anxiety. Sometimes used for premenstrual symptoms.

Dependency and Addiction: Do not stop taking buspirone without talking to your doctor, especially if you have taken large doses for a long time. Your doctor probably will decrease your dose gradually.

Withdrawals:

Abdominal cramps
Agitation (suddenly violent and forceful, emotionally disturbed state of mind)
Anxiety
Flu-like symptoms without fever
Insomnia
Irrtability
Muscle cramps
Seizures (occasionally)
Sweating
Vomiting

Important Warnings:

Patients should be cautioned about operating an automobile or using heavy or complex machinery until they are reasonably certain that buspirone does not affect them adversely.

The more commonly observed adverse events associated with the use of BuSpar include
Dizziness
Excitement
Headache
Light-headedness
Nervousness

Brand Name: Celexa
Generic Name: citaopram

Type or Class of Drug: Antidepressant

Approved for: Treatment of depression. Sometimes used to treat alcoholism, panic and eating problems.

Dependency and Addiction: Do not stop taking Celexa suddenly. If you do you may experience withdrawal symptoms.

If intolerable symptoms occur following a decrease in dose or upon stopping altogether then a doctor will likely have the patient go back to taking the previous dose and then try reducing the dosage again, this time more gradually.

Withdrawals:

Agitation (suddenly violent and forceful, emotionally disturbed state of mind)
Anxiety
Confusion
Difficulty falling asleep
Difficulty staying asleep
Disturbance of the senses such as electric shock sensations
Dizziness
Dysphoria (anxiety, depression ,unease)
Emotional lability (excessive emotional reactions and frequent mood changes.)
Headache
Hypomania (a state of mind and mood where a person may have excessive energy, little need for sleep, unusual exhilaration, irritability, excitement or aggression)
Insomnia
Irritability
Lethargy
Mood changes
Numbness or tingling in the hands or feet
Parethesias (Paresthesia is a skin sensation such as burning, prickling, itching or tingling with no physical cause. It could be temporary or permanent.)
Tiredness

Important Warnings: The Black Box Label placed by the FDA on antidepressants including Celexa includes an extensive list of serious, life-threatening potential consequences. There is a tendency among medical professionals and of course with the pharmaceutical and psychiatric industry to downplay these warnings. Don't be fooled. These are real. They do happen and have happened to real people. The FDA does not place warnings like these lightly.

This Black Box Label includes the following warnings. Note that this is not the complete Black Box Label. That can be found at the FDA MedlinePlus website listed in the resources section at the end of this booklet.

* Children, teenagers, and young adults who take antidepressants to treat depression or other mental illnesses may be more likely to become suicidal than children, teenagers, and young adults who do not take antidepressants to treat these conditions.

* You should know that your mental health may change in unexpected ways when you take citalopram or other antidepressants even if you are an adult over 24 years of age. You may become suicidal, especially at the beginning of your treatment and any time that your dose is increased or decreased.

* You, your family, or your caregiver should call your doctor right away if you experience any of the following symptoms: Make sure someone around you such as a family member or friend or caregiver knows these symptoms so they can call the doctor if you are unable to seek treatment on your own.

Acting without thinking
Aggressive behavior
Agitation (suddenly violent and forceful, emotionally disturbed state of mind)
Difficulty falling asleep
Difficulty staying asleep
Extreme worry
Frenzied abnormal excitement
Irritability
New or worsening depression
Panic attacks
Planning to kill yourself
Severe restlessness
Thinking about harming yourself
Thinking about killing yourself
Trying to kill yourself

Brand Name: Concerta
Generic Name: methylphenidate

Type or Class of Drug: Central Nervous System Stimulant
[A stimulant is a drug that increases heart rate, breathing rate, brain function. And nervous system.]

Approved for: ADHD and Narcolepsy

Dependency and Addiction: Methylphenidate can be habit-forming. Methylphenidate can be habit-forming. Do not take a larger dose, take it more often, take it for a longer time, or take it in a different way than prescribed by your doctor. If you take too much methylphenidate, you may find that the medication no longer controls your symptoms, you may feel a need to take large amounts of the medication, and you may experience unusual changes in your behavior

Withdrawals:

Do not stop taking methylphenidate without talking to your doctor. The main withdrawal symptoms noted are:

Severe depression
Extreme fatigue
Changes in heart rhythm.

Important Warnings:

Methylphenidate may cause sudden death in children and teenagers, especially children or teenagers with heart defects or serious heart problems.

This medication also may cause sudden death, heart attack or stroke in adults, especially adults with heart defects or serious heart problems.

Methylphenidate may slow children's growth or weight gain.

Stimulants such as Concerta create a rise in blood pressure.

Stimulants may make any problems with behavior or problems a person is having with their thoughts worse than they were before taking the medication.

Aggressive behavior or hostility has been seen in connection with the taking of stimulants. This behavior should be watched for in patients taking Concerta.

Psychotic and manic symptoms such as hallucinations or delusional thinking can be caused by this drug in patients who have had not previous history of these feelings and problems. This can occur at just normal doses prescribed by a doctor.

Difficulty focusing and blurring of vision have been reported in people taking stimulant drugs such as Concerta.

There is some evidence stimulants may cause seizures.

Other adverse reactions to stimulants include:

Anxiety
Blood pressure increased
Decreased appetite
Dizziness
Dry mouth
Headache
Hyperhidrosis (excessive sweating)
Insomnia
Irritability
Nausea
Upper abdominal pain
Weight decreased

Brand Name: Cymbalta
Generic Name: duloxetine

Type or Class of Drug: Antidepressant

Approved for: Depression, Anxiety, fibromyalgia, diabetic neuropathy

Dependency and Addiction: Do not stop taking duloxetine without talking to your doctor. Your doctor will probably decrease your dose gradually. If you suddenly stop taking duloxetine, you may experience withdrawal symptoms

Withdrawals: Withdrawal symptoms include:

Anxiety
Burning, numbness or tingling in hands or feet
Diarrhea
Difficulty falling asleep
Difficulty staying asleep
Dizziness
Headache
Irritability
Sweating
Nausea
Nightmares
Pain
Tiredness
Vomiting

Important Warnings: The Black Box Label placed by the FDA on antidepressants including Cymbalta includes an extensive list of serious, life-threatening potential consequences. A tendency exists among medical professionals and of course with the pharmaceutical and psychiatric industry to downplay these warnings. Don't be fooled. These are real. They do happen and have happened to real people. The FDA does not place warnings like these lightly.

This Black Box Label includes the following warnings. Note that this is not the complete Black Box Label. That can be found at the FDA MedlinePlus website listed in the resources section at the end of this booklet.

Cymbalta is not approved for use in pediatric patients

A small number of children, teenagers, and young adults (up to 24 years of age) who took antidepressants ('mood elevators') such as duloxetine during clinical studies became suicidal (thinking about harming or killing oneself or planning or trying to do so).

Children, teenagers, and young adults who take antidepressants to treat depression or other mental illnesses may be more likely to become suicidal than children, teenagers, and young adults who do not take antidepressants to treat these conditions.

You should know that your mental health may change in unexpected ways when you take duloxetine or other antidepressants even if you are an adult over 24 years of age.

These changes may occur even if you do not have a mental illness and you are taking duloxetine to treat a different type of condition.

You may become suicidal taking this drug.

You, your family, or caregiver should call your doctor right away if you experience any of the following symptoms:

Acting without thinking
Aggressive behavior
Agitation (suddenly violent and forceful, emotionally disturbed state of mind)
Behavior changes (any other unusual changes in behavior)
Difficulty falling asleep
Difficulty staying asleep
Extreme worry
Frenzied, abnormal excitement
Hostile behavior
Irritability
New or worsening depression

Panic attacks
Planning or trying to kill yourself
Severe restlessness
Thinking about harming yourself
Thinking about killing yourself

Be sure that your family or caregiver checks on you daily so they can call the doctor if you are unable to seek treatment on your own.

Brand Name: Dalmane
Generic Name: flurazepam

Type or Class of Drug: Benzodiazepine - Minor Sedative
(A benzodiazepine is one of the types of drugs used as tranquilizers or sedatives or hypnotics or muscle relaxants; chronic use can lead to dependency)

Approved for: Treatment of Insomnia

Dependency and Addiction: Flurazepam can be habit-forming. Do not take a larger dose, take it more often, or take it for a longer time than prescribed by your doctor.
May produce psychological and physical dependence, it is advisable that they consult with their physician before either increasing the dose or abruptly discontinuing this drug.

Withdrawals: If you suddenly stop taking flurazepam, especially after taking it regularly, you may develop withdrawal symptoms such as:

Difficulty sleeping
Muscle cramps
Sadness
Seizures
Stomach cramps
Sweating
Uncontrollable shaking of part of your body
Vomiting

Important Warnings:

This has not been tested and is not recommended for use in children.

Complex behaviors such as "sleep-driving" (i.e., driving while not fully awake after ingestion of a sedative-hypnotic, with amnesia for the event) have been reported.

Other complex behaviors (e.g., preparing and eating food, making phone calls, or having sex) have been reported in patients who are not fully awake after taking a sedative-hypnotic. As with sleep-driving, patients usually do not remember these events.

Patients should also be cautioned about engaging in hazardous occupations requiring complete mental alertness such as operating machinery or driving a motor vehicle after ingesting the drug, including potential impairment of the performance of such activities which may occur the day following ingestion of Flurazepam Hydrochloride Capsules.

Warning for the elderly and debilitated: Dizziness, drowsiness, light-headedness, staggering, ataxia and falling have occurred, particularly in elderly or debilitated persons

Severe sedation, lethargy, disorientation and coma, probably indicative of drug intolerance or overdosage, have been reported.

Other Adverse Reactions that have been reported are:

Anorexia (loss of appetite especially as result of disease)
Apprehension (Fearful or uneasy anticipation of the future; dread.)
Blurred vision
Body and joint pains
Burning vision
Chest pains
Confusion
Constipation
Depression
Diarrhea
Difficulty focusing
Dry mouth

Euphoria
Excessive salivation
Faintness
Flushing
Gastrointestinal pain (affecting the stomach and intestines)
Genitourinary complaints (of or relating to the genital and urinary organs or their functions.)
Headache
Heartburn
Hallucinations
Hypotension (low blood pressure)
Irritability
Nausea
Nervousness
Palpitations (heartbeat sensations that feel like your heart is pounding or racing)
Pruritus (severe itching, often of normal skin)
Restlessness
Shortness of breath
Skin rash
Slurred speech
Sweating
Talkativeness
Upset stomach
Vomiting
Weakness

Brand: Darvocet
Generic: Acetaminophen and Propoxyphene

Type or Class of Drug: Pain Reliever - Opioid
A narcotic is a substance that dulls pain and induces sleep. Opiate or opioid means that is derived from or acts like opium in dulling the senses and inducing sleep.

Approved for: Treat mild to moderate pain, treat fever

Dependency and Addiction: This drug can be habit-forming. Do not take a larger dose, take it more often, or for a longer period than your doctor tells you to. Should not be abruptly discontinued.

Withdrawals: Withdrawal symptoms for Darvocet include some or all of the following:

Abdominal cramps
Anorexia (loss of appetite especially as result of disease)
Anxiety
Backache
Chills
Diarrhea
Increased blood pressure
Increased heart rate
Increased respiratory rate
Insomnia
Irritability
Joint pain
Myalgia (muscular pain or tenderness)
Mydriasis (prolonged and abnormal dilation (expanding, getting larger) of the pupil often due to drugs)
Nausea
Restlessness
Runny nose
Sweating
Vomiting
Watery eyes
Weakness
Yawning

Important Warnings:

There have been numerous cases of accidental and intentional overdose connected with Darvocet alone or in combination with other drugs.

Do not take Darvocet (propoxyphene) in combination with other drugs that cause drowsiness: alcohol, tranquilizers, sleep aids, antidepressant drugs, or antihistamines.

Fatalities within the first hour of over-dosage are not uncommon.

Should not be prescribed for patients who are suicidal or have a history of suicidal ideation.

May cause high blood pressure.

May cause respiratory depression especially in the elderly and the debilitated. (respiratory depression is breathing that is slower than normal or which fails to fill the lungs as well as normal)

During the clinical trials where this drug was tested the reported adverse reactions included:

Abdominal pain
Constipation
Dizziness
Dysphoria (a state of anxiety, depression , unease)
Euphoria
Hallucinations (Seeing or hearing things that aren't there)
Headache
Lightheadedness
Minor visual disturbances
Nausea
Sedation
Skin rashes
Vomiting
Weakness

Since Darvocet has been on the market the most frequently reported adverse events have included:

Accidental overdose
Cardiac arrest
Cardio-respiratory arrest
Coma
Completed suicide
Confusional state
Convulsions

Death
Diarrhea
Dizziness
Drug dependence
Drug ineffective
Drug toxicity
Intentional overdose
Nausea
Respiratory arrest
Vomiting

Opioid painkillers now cause more drug overdose deaths than cocaine and heroin combined.

Brand: Darvon
Generic: propoxyphene

Type or Class of Drug: Pain Reliever - opioid
A narcotic is a substance that dulls pain and induces sleep. Opiate means that is derived from or acts like opium in dulling the senses and inducing sleep.

Approved for: Treat mild to moderate pain

Dependency and Addiction: This drug can be habit-forming. Do not take a larger dose, take it more often, or for a longer period than your doctor tells you to. Should not be abruptly discontinued.

Withdrawals: Withdrawal symptoms for Darvon include some or all of the following:

Abdominal cramps
Anorexia (loss of appetite especially as result of disease)
Anxiety
Backache

Chills
Diarrhea
Increased blood pressure
Increased heart rate
Increased respiratory rate
Insomnia
Irritability
Joint pain
Myalgia (muscular pain or tenderness)
Mydriasis (prolonged and abnormal dilation (expanding, getting larger) of the pupil often due to drugs)
Nausea
Restlessness
Runny nose
Sweating
Vomiting
Watery eyes
Weakness
Yawning

Important Warnings:

There have been numerous cases of accidental and intentional overdose connected with Darvon alone or in combination with other drugs.

Do not take Darvon (propoxyphene) in combination with other drugs that cause drowsiness: alcohol, tranquilizers, sleep aids, antidepressant drugs, or antihistamines.

Fatalities within the first hour of over-dosage are not uncommon.

Patients should be advised that Darvon may impair mental and/or physical ability required for the performance of potentially hazardous tasks (e.g., driving, operating heavy machinery).

Should not be prescribed for patients who are suicidal or have a history of suicidal ideation.

May cause high blood pressure.

May cause respiratory depression especially in the elderly and the debilitated. (respiratory depression is breathing that is slower than normal or which fails to fill the lungs as well as normal)

During the clinical trials where this drug was tested the reported adverse reactions included:

Abdominal pain
Constipation
Dizziness
Dysphoria (a state of anxiety, depression ,unease)
Euphoria
Hallucinations
Headache
Lightheadedness
Minor visual disturbances
Nausea
Sedation
Skin rashes
Vomiting
Weakness

Since propoxyphene (Darvon) has been on the market the most frequently reported adverse events have included:

Accidental overdose
Cardiac arrest
Cardio-respiratory arrest
Coma
Completed suicide
Confusional state
Convulsions
Death
Diarrhea
Dizziness
Drug dependence
Drug ineffective
Drug toxicity

Intentional overdose
Nausea
Respiratory arrest
Vomiting

Opioid painkillers now cause more drug overdose deaths than cocaine and heroin combined.

Brand Name: Demerol
Generic Name: meperidine

Type or Class of Drug: Narcotic pain reliever (a group of pain medications similar to morphine)

Approved for: Relieve moderate to severe pain

Dependency and Addiction: Meperidine can be habit-forming. Do not take a larger dose, or take it more often or for a longer period of time than you were told by your doctor. Your doctor will want to reduce your dosage gradually.

Withdrawals: Withdrawal symptoms may include:

Abdominal cramps
Anorexia (loss of appetite especially as result of disease)
Anxiety
Back pain
Chills
Diarrhea
Fast breathing
Fast heart rate
Increased blood pressure
Increased heart rate
Increased respiratory rate
Insomnia
Irritability
Joint pain
Loss of appetite
Muscle pain

Myalgia (muscular pain or tenderness)
Mydriasis (prolonged and abnormal dilation (expanding, getting larger) of the pupil often due to drugs)
Nausea
Nervousness
Restlessness
Stomach pain
Stuffy nose
Sweating
Upset stomach
Vomiting
Watery eyes
Weakness
Yawning

Important Warnings:

Alcohol and street drugs can make the side effects from meperidine worse and can cause serious harm or death.

Do not drive a car or operate machinery until you know how this medication affects you.

The major hazards of meperidine are:

Cardiac arrest
Circulatory depression
Respiratory arrest
Respiratory depression (trouble breathing)
Shock

The most frequently observed adverse reactions include:

Dizziness
Lightheadedness
Nausea
Sedation
Sweating
Vomiting

Brand Name: Desyrel
Generic Name: trazodone

Type or Class of Drug: Antidepressant

Approved for: Trazodone is used to treat depression. Sometimes prescribed for insomnia and schizophrenia.

Dependency and Addiction: None mentioned in labeling. However, do not stop taking without checking with your doctor.

Withdrawals: Do not stop taking trazodone without talking to your doctor. Your doctor will probably decrease your dose gradually.

Important Warnings:

The Black Box Label placed by the FDA on antidepressants including Cymbalta includes an extensive list of serious, life-threatening potential consequences. There is a tendency among medical professionals and of course with the pharmaceutical and psychiatric industry to downplay these warnings. Don't be fooled. These are real. They do happen and have happened to real people. The FDA does not place warnings like these lightly.

This Black Box Label includes the following warnings. Note that this is not the complete Black Box Label. That can be found at the FDA MedlinePlus website listed in the resources section at the end of this booklet.

Cymbalta is not approved for use in pediatric patients

A small number of children, teenagers, and young adults (up to 24 years of age) who took antidepressants ('mood elevators') such as duloxetine during clinical studies became suicidal (thinking about harming or killing oneself or planning or trying to do so).

Children, teenagers, and young adults who take antidepressants to treat depression or other mental illnesses may be more likely to become suicidal than children, teenagers, and young adults who do not take antidepressants to treat these conditions.

You should know that your mental health may change in unexpected ways when you take duloxetine or other antidepressants even if you are an adult over 24 years of age.

These changes may occur even if you do not have a mental illness and you are taking duloxetine to treat a different type of condition.

You may become suicidal taking this drug.

You, your family, or caregiver should call your doctor right away if you experience any of the following symptoms:

Acting without thinking
Aggressive behavior
Agitation (suddenly violent and forceful, emotionally disturbed state of mind)
Behavior changes (any other unusual changes in behavior)
Difficulty falling asleep
Difficulty staying asleep
Extreme worry
Frenzied, abnormal excitement
Hostile behavior
Irritability
New or worsening depression
Panic attacks
Planning or trying to kill yourself
Severe restlessness
Thinking about harming yourself
Thinking about killing yourself

Be sure that your family or caregiver checks on you daily so they can call the doctor if you are unable to seek treatment on your own.

Trazodone may cause painful, long lasting erections in males. In some cases emergency and/or surgical treatment has been required and, in some of these cases, permanent damage has occurred

Brand Name: Dexedrine
Generic Name: Dextroamphentamine

Type or Class of Drug: Central Nervous System Stimulant
[A stimulant is a drug that increases heart rate, breathing rate, brain function. And nervous system.]

Approved for: ADHD, Narcolepsy

Dependency and Addiction: Dextroamphetamine can be habit-forming. Do not take a larger dose, take it more often, or take it for a longer time than prescribed by your doctor. If you take too much dextroamphetamine you may find that the medication no longer controls your symptoms, you may feel a need to take large amounts of the medication.

Do not stop taking dextroamphetamine without talking to your doctor.

Your doctor will probably decrease your dose gradually and monitor you carefully during this time.

Withdrawals:

You may experience depression and extreme tiredness if you suddenly stop taking dextroamphetamine after overusing it.

Important Warnings:

If you take a larger dose or take this drug more frequently than you should you may experience the following (Be alert to the following in your or someone you love even if this drug is being taken as prescribed.)

Difficulty falling asleep
Difficulty staying asleep
Hyperactivity (a condition characterized by excessive restlessness and movement)

Rash
Unusual changes in your behavior
Unusual changes in your personality

Overusing dextroamphetamine may also cause serious heart problems or sudden death.

Dextroamphetamine may slow children's growth or weight gain.

Dextroamphetamine may cause sudden death in children and teenagers, especially children and teenagers with heart defects or serious heart problems.

Dextroamphetamine may cause sudden death, heart attack, or stroke in adults, especially adults who have heart defects or other serious heart problems.

Amphetamines may impair your ability to engage in potentially hazardous activities such as operating machinery or vehicles.

Amphetamines are excreted in human milk. Mothers taking amphetamines should be advised to refrain from nursing.

The following have been reported with use of DEXEDRINE and other stimulant medicines:

Sudden death in patients who have had heart problems and heart defects
Stroke and heart attack in adults
Increased blood pressure and heart rate
New or worse behavior and thought problems (applies to all ages)
New or worse bipolar illness (applies to all ages)
New or worse aggressive behavior or hostility (applies to all ages)
Psychotic symptoms in children and teenagers such as hearing voices, believing things that are not true
New manic behavior (mania is defined as abnormally and persistently elevated, expansive, or irritable mood)

Call your doctor right away if you or your child have any new or worsening mental symptoms or problems while taking

DEXEDRINE, especially seeing or hearing things that are not real, believing things that are not real, or are suspicious.

Brand Name: Dilaudid
Generic Name: hydromorphone

Type or Class of Drug: Pain reliever

Approved for: Relieve moderate to severe pain. May also be used to decrease coughing.

Dependancy and Addiction: Hydromorphone can be habit-forming. Do not take a larger dose, take it more often, or for a longer period than your doctor tells you to.

Withdrawals: Physical dependence results in withdrawal symptoms in patients who abruptly discontinue the drug. Withdrawal symptoms include:

Abdominal cramps
Acute withdrawal syndrome
Anorexia (loss of appetite especially as result of disease)
Anxiety
Backache
Chills
Diarrhea
Increased blood pressure
Increased heart rate
Increased respiratory rate
Insomnia
Irritability
Joint pain
Myalgia (muscular pain or tenderness)
Mydriasis (prolonged and abnormal dilation (expanding, getting larger) of the pupil often due to drugs)
Perspiration
Restlessness
Runny nose
Vomiting
Watery eyes

Weakness
Yawning

Important Warnings:

Infants born to mothers physically dependent on Dilaudid will also be physically dependent and may exhibit respiratory difficulties and withdrawal symptoms.

Adverse reactions to this drug include:

The major hazards of Dilauded are respiratory depression and apnea (breathing that slows or stops from any cause).

Other hazards include:

Cardiac arrest
Circulatory depression
Dizziness
Dry mouth
Dysphoria (a state of anxiety, depression ,unease)
Euphoria
Flushing
Light-headedness
Nausea
Pruritus
Respiratory arrest
Sedation
Shock
Sweating
Vomiting

Risk of respiratory depression that might result in death

Brand Name: Duragesic
Generic Name: fentanyl

Type or Class of Drug: Pain reliever

Approved for: Relieve moderate to severe pain that are expected to last for some time

Dependancy and Addiction: Fentanyl skin patches may be habit forming. Do not apply more than one patch at a time unless your doctor tells you that you should, and do not apply fentanyl skin patches more often, or for a longer period of time than prescribed by your doctor.

Withdrawals:

Withdrawal syndrome is characterized by some or all of the following:
Abdominal cramps
Anxiety
Backache
Chills
Diarrhea
Difficulty falling asleep
Difficulty staying asleep
Hair standing on end
Increased blood pressure
Increased heart rate
Increased respiratory rate
Insomnia
Irritability
Joint pain
Large pupils
Loss of appetite
Muscle aches
Myalgia
Mydriasis
Nausea
Perspiration
Piloerection

Restlessness
Runny nose
Stomach cramps
Sweating
Vomiting
Watery eyes
Weakness
Yawning

Important Warnings:

Anytime you are prescribed a medication by your doctor make sure you tell her or him about all other prescribed and over-the-counter medications you are taking as well as any vitamins, herbs or other supplements.

Fentanyl skin patches should not be used to treat mild pain, short-term pain, pain after an operation or medical or dental procedure, or pain that can be controlled by medication that is taken as needed.

Fentanyl skin patches may cause serious or life-threatening breathing problems, especially during the first 72 hours of your treatment.

Brand Name: Effexor / Effexor XR
Generic Name: venlafaxine

Type or Class of Drug: Antidepressant

Approved for: Depression, anxiety, panic, hot flashes

Dependancy and Addiction: Your doctor will probably decrease your dose gradually. If you suddenly stop taking venlafaxine, you may experience withdrawal symptoms. Tell your doctor if you experience any of the following no matter whether you are tapering off Effexor or not.

Withdrawals: Withdrawal symptoms include:

Abnormal excitement
Agitation (suddenly violent and forceful, emotionally disturbed state of mind)
Anorexia (loss of appetite especially as result of disease)
Anxiety
Burning like feelings in any part of the body
Confusion
Diarrhea
Dizziness
Dry mouth
Electric shock like feelings in any part of the body
Fatigue
Frenzied excitement
Irritability
Lack of coordination
Loss of appetite
Nausea
Nightmares
Numbness in any part of the body
Ringing in the ears
Sad mood
Seizures
Sweating
Tingling in any part of the body
Tinnitus
Trouble falling asleep
Trouble staying asleep
Vertigo
Vomiting

Important Warnings: Effexor and Effexor XR have many warnings including the FDA's Black Box Warning. These warnings include:

Any psychoactive drug including Effexor may impair judgment, thinking, or motor skills

Antidepressants increased the risk of suicidal thinking and behavior (suicidality) in children, adolescents, and young adults.

Your mental health may change in unexpected ways when you take Effexor (venlafaxine) or other antidepressants even if you are an adult over 24 years of age.

You may become suicidal on this medication.

Patients, their families, and their caregivers should be encouraged to be alert to the emergence of the following symptoms in patients taking Effexor or Effexor XR:

Aggressiveness
Agitation (suddenly violent and forceful, emotionally disturbed state of mind)
Akathisia (A state of restlessness ranging from a feeling of inner distress to an inability to sit still)
Anxiety
Hostility
Hypomania (persistent and pervasive elated or irritable mood, and thoughts and behaviors)
Impulsivity
Insomnia
Irritability
Other unusual changes in behavior
Panic attacks
Suicidal ideation
Worsening of depression

Families and caregivers of patients should be advised to look for the emergence of such symptoms on a day-to-day basis, since changes may be abrupt.

Brand Name: Halcion
Generic Name: triazolam

Type or Class of Drug: Benzodiazepine - sedative
(Benzodiazepine is one of the types of drugs used as tranquilizers or sedatives or hypnotics or muscle relaxants; chronic use can lead to dependency)

Approved for: Used to treat insomnia on a short-term basis

Dependancy and Addiction: There can be severe 'withdrawal' effects when a benzodiazepine sleeping pill is stopped.

Withdrawals: Such effects can occur after discontinuing these drugs following use for only a week or two, but may be more common and more severe after longer periods of continuous use.

Withdrawals may include:

Abdominal cramps
Convulsions (rarely)
Dysphoria (a state of anxiety, depression, unease)
Increased signs of daytime anxiety or nervousness
Mild unpleasant feelings
Muscle cramps
Perceptual disturbances
Rebound insomnia (insomnia worse than it was before)
Sweating
Tremors
Vomiting

Important Warnings:

You will probably become very sleepy soon after you take triazolam and will remain sleepy for some time after you take the medication. Plan to go to bed right after you take triazolam and to stay in bed for 7 to 8 hours. Do not take triazolam if you will be unable to remain asleep for 7 to 8 hours after taking the medication.

If you get up too soon after taking triazolam, you may experience memory problems.

Tell your doctor right away if you experience any of the following symptoms:
Aggressiveness
Confusion
Difficulty concentrating
Feeling like you are outside of your body

Hallucinations (seeing things or hearing voices that do not exist)
Memory problems
New depression
Slowed movements
Slowed speech
Strange or unusually outgoing behavior
Suicidal thoughts (thinking about killing yourself)
Worsening depression

Any other changes in your thoughts, mood or behavior.

Be sure that your family knows about these symptoms so that they can call the doctor if you are unable to seek treatment on your own.

An increase in daytime anxiety has been reported for Halcion after as few as 10 days of continuous use.

Brand Name: Haldol
Generic Name: haloperidol

Type or Class of Drug: antipsychotic

Approved for: Used to treat psychotic disorders, Tourette's disorder, severe behavioral problems such as explosive, aggressive behavior or hyperactivity in children who cannot be treated with psychotherapy or with other medications

Dependancy and Addiction: Your doctor will probably decrease your dose gradually. If you suddenly stop taking haloperidol, you may experience difficulty controlling your movements.

Withdrawals: If you suddenly stop taking haloperidol, you may experience difficulty controlling your movements.

Important Warnings:

Tardive dyskinesia, a syndrome consisting of potentially irreversible, involuntary, dyskinetic movements, may appear in some patients on long-term therapy or may occur after drug therapy has been discontinued. The syndrome is characterized by rhythmical involuntary movements of tongue, face, mouth or jaw (e.g., protrusion of tongue, puffing of cheeks, puckering of mouth, chewing movements). Sometimes these may be accompanied by involuntary movements of extremities and the trunk.

The following have been reported in connection with taking Haldol:

Agitation (suddenly violent and forceful, emotionally disturbed state of mind)
Anxiety
Catatonic-like behavior (Behavior characterized by muscular tightness or rigidity and lack of response to the environment.)
Confusion
Depression
Drowsiness
Euphoria
Gand mal seizures (a violent seizure involving the entire body)
Hallucinations
Headache
Insomnia
Lethargy
Restlessness
Worsening of psychotic symptoms

May cause heart failure or sudden death.

Treatment with antipsychotic drugs may increase mortality.

Brand Name: Klonopin
Generic Name: clonazepam

Type or Class of Drug: benzodiazepine (one of the types of drugs used as tranquilizers or sedatives or hypnotics or muscle relaxants; chronic use can lead to dependency)

Approved for: To control certain types of seizures, treat panic attacks

Dependency and Addiction: Clonazepam can be habit-forming. Do not take a larger dose, take it more often, or take it for a longer period of time or in a different way than prescribed by your doctor.

Withdrawals: Your doctor will probably decrease your dose gradually.

If you suddenly stop taking clonazepam, you may experience withdrawal symptoms such as:
Anxiety
Changes in behavior
Difficulty falling asleep
Difficulty staying asleep
Hallucinating (seeing things or hearing voices that do not exist)
Muscle cramps
New seizures
Stomach cramps
Sweating
Uncontrollable shaking of a part of your body
Worsening seizures

Important Warnings:

May increase mortality

Cases of sudden death have been reported.

You should know that your mental health may change in unexpected ways, and you may become suicidal (thinking about harming or killing yourself or planning or trying to do so) while you are taking clonazepam

You, your family, or your caregiver should call your doctor right away if you experience any of the following symptoms:

Acting on dangerous impulses
Aggressive behavior
Agitation (suddenly violent and forceful, emotionally disturbed state of mind)
Angry behavior
Anxiety
Any other unusual changes in behavior or mood
Depression
Difficulty falling asleep
Difficulty staying asleep
Giving away prized possessions
Irritability
Mania (frenzied, abnormally excited mood)
New Irritability
Panic attacks
Preoccupation with death or dying
Restlessness
Talking or thinking about wanting to end your life
Talking or thinking about wanting to hurt yourself
Violent behavior
Withdrawing from friends or family
Worsening irritability

Be sure that your family or caregiver knows these symptoms so they can call the doctor if you are unable to seek treatment on your own.

Brand Name: Lexapro
Generic Name: escitalopram

Type or Class of Drug: Antidepressant

Approved for: Treatment of depression, treatment of anxiety

Dependency and Addiction: Do not stop taking escitalopram without talking to your doctor. If you suddenly stop taking escitalopram, you may experience withdrawal symptoms.

Withdrawals:

Agitation (suddenly violent and forceful, emotionally disturbed state of mind)
Anxiety
Confusion
Difficulty falling asleep
Difficulty staying asleep
Dizziness
Headache
Irritability
Mood changes
Numbness in hands or feet
Tingling in hands or feet
Tiredness

Important Warnings:

The Black Box Label placed by the FDA on antidepressants including Lexapro includes an extensive list of serious, life-threatening potential consequences. There is a tendency among medical professionals and of course with the pharmaceutical and psychiatric industry to downplay these warnings. Don't be fooled. These are real. They do happen and have happened to real people. The FDA does not place warnings like these lightly.

This Black Box Label includes the following warnings. Note that this is not the complete Black Box Label. That can be found at the FDA MedlinePlus website listed in the resources section at the end of this booklet.

* Children, teenagers, and young adults who take antidepressants to treat depression or other mental illnesses may be more likely to become suicidal than children, teenagers, and young adults who do not take antidepressants to treat these conditions.

* You should know that your mental health may change in unexpected ways when you take citalopram or other antidepressants even if you are an adult over 24 years of age. You may become suicidal, especially at the beginning of your treatment and any time that your dose is increased or decreased.

* You, your family, or your caregiver should call your doctor right away if you experience any of the following symptoms: Make sure someone around you such as a family member or friend or caregiver knows these symptoms so they can call the doctor if you are unable to seek treatment on your own.

Acting without thinking
Aggressive behavior
Agitation (suddenly violent and forceful, emotionally disturbed state of mind)
Difficulty falling asleep
Difficulty staying asleep
Extreme worry
Frenxied abnormal excitement
Irritability
New or worsening depression
Panic attacks
Planning to kill yourself
Severe restlessness
Thinking about harming yourself
Thinking about killing yourself
Trying to kill yourself

Brand Name: Librium
Generic Name: chlordiazepoxide

Type or Class of Drug: Benzodiazepine - minor sedative
(One of the types of drugs used as tranquilizers or sedatives or hypnotics or muscle relaxants; chronic use can lead to dependency)

Approved for: Treatment of anxiety, to control agitation caused by alcohol withdrawal, also used to treat irritable bowel syndrome

Dependency and Addiction: Chlordiazepoxide can be habit-forming. Do not take a larger dose, take it more often, or for a longer time than your doctor tells you to. Tolerance may develop with long-term or excessive use, making the drug less effective.

Withdrawals: Stopping the drug suddenly can worsen your condition and cause withdrawal symptoms such as:

Abdominal cramps
Anxiousness
Convulsions
Dysphoria (a state of anxiety, depression, unease)
Insomnia
Irritability
Muscle cramps
Sleeplessness
Sweating
Tremor
Vomiting

Important Warnings:

In addition to the side effects, precautions and warnings shown on the label the following have been reported:

Ataxia (Loss of the ability to coordinate muscular movement)
Confusion
Drowsiness

Brand Name: Lorcet
Generic Name: hydrocodone and acetaminophen

Type or Class of Drug: Opiate (narcotic) pain killer
A narcotic is a substance that dulls pain and induces sleep. Opiate means that is derived from or acts like opium in dulling the senses and inducing sleep.

Approved for: Treatment of pain and coughing

Dependency and Addiction: Hydrocodone may be habit-forming. Take hydrocodone exactly as directed. Do not take a larger dose, take it more often, or take it for a longer period of time than prescribed by your doctor. Call your doctor if you develop a strong desire to take more medication than prescribed.

The acetaminophen part of this drug is not habit forming however it does have side effects and serious overdose cautions. Please see FDA MedlinePlus web site referenced at the end of this booklet for more information.

Withdrawals: If you suddenly stop taking hydrocodone, you may experience withdrawal symptoms.

Anxiety
Back pain
Chills
Cravings
Depression
Diarrhea
Fatigue
Feeling sick
Flu-like symptoms
Insomnia
Irritability
Loss of apetite
Muscle aches
Muscle pains
Runny nose
Sleep disturbances
Sweating
Watery eyes
Yawning

Important Warnings:

"Doctor shopping" to obtain additional prescriptions is common among drug abusers and people suffering from untreated addiction.

Call your doctor if your symptoms are not controlled by the hydrocodone product you are taking. Do not increase your dose of medication on your own.

Hydrocodone may make you drowsy. Do not drive a car or operate machinery until you know how this medication affects you.

Brand Name: Lomotil
Generic Name: diohenoxylate and atropine

Type or Class of Drug: Antidiarrhea

Approved for: Lomotril (Diphenoxylate and atropine) is used to control diarrhea.

Dependency and Addiction: Diphenoxylate can be habit-forming. Do not take a larger dose, take it more often, or for a longer period than your doctor tells you to. Stopping the medicine suddenly after taking it for a long time may cause withdrawal.

Withdrawals:

Muscle cramps
Shaking
Stomach cramps
Trembling
Unusual sweating
Upset stomach
Vomiting

Important Warnings:

You should know that this drug may make you drowsy. Do not drive a car or operate machinery until you know how this drug affects you.

Brand Name: Lunesta
Generic Name: eszopiclone

Type or Class of Drug: Hypnotic

Approved for: Insomnia

Dependency and Addiction: Do not stop taking eszopiclone without talking to your doctor. Your doctor will probably decrease your dose gradually

Withdrawals: . If you suddenly stop taking eszopiclone you may experience withdrawal symptoms such as:

Anxiety
Muscle cramps
Seizures (rarely)
Shakiness
Stomach cramps
Sweating
Unusual dreams
Vomiting

Important Warnings:

Your mental health may change in unexpected ways

Tell your doctor right away if you experience any of the following symptoms:
Aggressiveness
Confusion
Feeling as if you are outside of your body
Hallucinations (seeing things or hearing voices that do not exist)
Memory problems
New depression
Other unusual behavior
Other unusual thoughts
Strange or unusually outgoing behavior
Thinking about killing yourself
Worsening depression

Be sure that your family knows these symptoms so that they can call the doctor if you are unable to seek treatment on your own.

A variety of abnormal thinking and behavior changes have been reported to occur in association with the use of sedative/hypnotics.

Do not engage in hazardous occupations requiring complete mental alertness or motor coordination such as operating machinery or driving a motor vehicle after taking Lunesta. You may suffer these same problems the day after taking this drug.

Brand Name: Lyrica
Generic Name: pregabalin

Type or Class of Drug: Anticonvulsant

Approved for: To treat pain from damaged nerves if you have Diabetes. It is also used to treat pain from shingles and is used to treat certain types of epileptic seizures. Used to treat pain associated with fibromyalgia.

Dependency and Addiction: Pregabalin may be habit forming. Do not take a larger dose, take it more often, or take it for a longer period of time than prescribed by your doctor.

Withdrawals: If you suddenly stop taking pregabalin, you may experience withdrawal symptoms including:

Diarrhea
Headaches
Nausea
Seizures
Trouble falling alseep
Trouble staying asleep

Important Warnings:

Your mental health may change in unexpected ways and you may become suicidal from taking this medication.

You or your family or care giver should notify your doctor right away if you experience any of the following:

Acting on dangerous impulses
Aggressiveness
Agitation (suddenly violent and forceful, emotionally disturbed state of mind)
Anger
Anxiety
Depression
Difficulty falling asleep
Difficulty staying asleep
Giving away prized posessions
Mania (frenzied, abnormally excited mood);
New irritability
Panic attacks
Preoccupation with death and dying
Restlessness
Talking about wanting to hurt yourself or end your life
Thinking about wanting to hurt yourself or end your life
Thinking of killing yourself or planning to do so
Trying to kill yourself
Unusual changes in behavior or mood
Violent behavior
Withdrawing from friends and family
Worsening irritability

Be sure that your family or caregiver knows these symptoms so they can call the doctor if you are unable to seek treatment on your own.

Brand Name: Narvox
Generic Name: oxycodone and acetaminophen

Type or Class of Drug: Opiate (narcotic) pain killer
A narcotic is a substance that dulls pain and induces sleep. Opiate
means that is derived from or acts like opium in dulling the senses
and inducing sleep.

Approved for: Relief of moderate to severe pain

Dependency and Addiction: Oxycodone can be habit-forming. Do
not take a larger dose, take it more often, or take it for a longer
period of time than prescribed by your doctor. If you have been
taking oxycodone for more than a few days, do not stop taking
oxycodone suddenly.

Oxycodone can produce drug dependence of the morphine type and,
therefore, has the potential for being abused.

Withdrawals: If you stop taking this medication suddenly, you
may experience withdrawal symptoms such as:

Anxiety
Chills
Cramps
Depression
Diarrhea
Difficulty falling asleep
Difficulty staying asleep
Fast breathing
Fast heartbeat
Irritability
Joint aches or pains
Loss of appetite
Muscle aches or pains
Nausea
Restlessness
Runny nose
Sneezing
Sweating
Vomiting

Watery eyes
Weakness
Yawning

Call your doctor if you have any withdrawal symptoms when your dose is decreased or when you stop taking oxycodone.

Important Warnings:

You should know that this medication may make you drowsy. Do not drive a car, operate heavy machinery, or participate in any other possibly dangerous activities until you know how this medication affects you.

Oxycodone may cause dizziness, lightheadedness, and fainting when you get up too quickly from a lying position.

See label or MedlinePlus web site for the full list of side effects and other warnings.

Brand Name: Oxycontin
Generic Name: oxycodone

Type or Class of Drug: Opiate (narcotic) pain killer
A narcotic is a substance that dulls pain and induces sleep. Opiate means that is derived from or acts like opium in dulling the senses and inducing sleep.

Approved for: Relief of moderate to severe pain

Dependency and Addiction: Oxycodone can be habit-forming. Do not take a larger dose, take it more often, or take it for a longer period of time than prescribed by your doctor. If you have been taking oxycodone for more than a few days, do not stop taking oxycodone suddenly.

Oxycodone can produce drug dependence of the morphine type and, therefore, has the potential for being abused.

Withdrawals: If you stop taking this medication suddenly, you may experience withdrawal symptoms such as:

Anxiety
Chills
Cramps
Depression
Diarrhea
Difficulty falling asleep
Difficulty staying asleep
Fast breathing
Fast heartbeat
Irritability
Joint aches or pains
Loss of appetite
Muscle aches or pains
Nausea
Restlessness
Runny nose
Sneezing
Sweating
Vomiting
Watery eyes
Weakness
Yawning

Call your doctor if you have any withdrawal symptoms when your dose is decreased or when you stop taking oxycodone.

Important Warnings:

You should know that this medication may make you drowsy. Do not drive a car, operate heavy machinery, or participate in any other possibly dangerous activities until you know how this medication affects you.

Oxycodone may cause dizziness, lightheadedness, and fainting when you get up too quickly from a lying position.

See label or MedlinePlus web site for the full list of side effects and other warnings.

Oxycontin is one of the most abused drugs on the market.

Brand Name: Paxil
Generic Name: paroxetine

Type or Class of Drug: Antidepressant

Approved for: Used to treat depression, panic disorder (sudden, unexpected attacks of extreme fear and worry about these attacks), and social anxiety disorder (extreme fear of interacting with others or performing in front of others that interferes with normal life).

Paroxetine is also sometimes used to treat chronic headaches, tingling in the hands and feet caused by diabetes, and certain male sexual problems

Are also used to treat obsessive-compulsive disorder (bothersome thoughts that won't go away and the need to perform certain actions over and over), generalized anxiety disorder (GAD; excessive worrying that is difficult to control), and posttraumatic stress disorder (disturbing psychological symptoms that develop after a frightening experience). Paroxetine extended-release tablets are also used to treat premenstrual dysphoric disorder (PMDD, physical and psychological symptoms that occur before the onset of the menstrual period each month).

Dependency and Addiction: Do not stop taking paroxetine without talking to your doctor. Your doctor will probably decrease your dose gradually.

Withdrawals: If you suddenly stop taking paroxetine, you may experience withdrawal symptoms such as:

Abnormally excited mood
Anxiety
Confusion
Depression
Difficulty falling asleep
Difficulty staying asleep
Dizziness
Frenzied mood
Headache
Irritability
Mood changes
Nausea
Numbness in arms, legs, hands or feet
Sweating
Tingling in arms, legs, hands or feet
Tiredness
Unusual dreams

Tell your doctor if you experience any of these symptoms when your dose of paroxetine is decreased.

Important Warnings:

The Black Box Label placed by the FDA on antidepressants including Paxil includes an extensive list of serious, life-threatening potential consequences. There is a tendency among medical professionals and of course with the pharmaceutical and psychiatric industry to downplay these warnings. Don't be fooled. These are real. They do happen and have happened to real people. The FDA does not place warnings like these lightly.

This Black Box Label includes the following warnings. Note that this is not the complete Black Box Label. That can be found at the FDA MedlinePlus website listed in the resources section at the end of this booklet.

* Children, teenagers, and young adults who take antidepressants to treat depression or other mental illnesses may be more likely to become suicidal than children, teenagers, and young adults who do not take antidepressants to treat these conditions.

* You should know that your mental health may change in unexpected ways when you take citalopram or other antidepressants even if you are an adult over 24 years of age. You may become suicidal, especially at the beginning of your treatment and any time that your dose is increased or decreased.

* You, your family, or your caregiver should call your doctor right away if you experience any of the following symptoms: Make sure someone around you such as a family member or friend or caregiver knows these symptoms so they can call the doctor if you are unable to seek treatment on your own.

Acting without thinking
Aggressive behavior
Agitation (suddenly violent and forceful, emotionally disturbed state of mind)
Difficulty falling asleep
Difficulty staying asleep
Extreme worry
Frenxied abnormal excitement
Irritability
New or worsening depression
Panic attacks
Planning to kill yourself
Severe restlessness
Thinking about harming yourself
Thinking about killing yourself
Trying to kill yourself

May make you drowsy and affect your judgment and thinking.

Brand Name: Percocet
Generic Name: oxycodone and acetaminophen

Type or Class of Drug: Opiate (narcotic) pain killer
A narcotic is a substance that dulls pain and induces sleep. Opiate means that is derived from or acts like opium in dulling the senses and inducing sleep.

Approved for: Relief of moderate to severe pain

Dependency and Addiction: Oxycodone can be habit-forming. Do not take a larger dose, take it more often, or take it for a longer period of time than prescribed by your doctor. If you have been taking oxycodone for more than a few days, do not stop taking oxycodone suddenly.

Oxycodone can produce drug dependence of the morphine type and, therefore, has the potential for being abused.

The acetaminophen part of this drug is not habit forming however it does have side effects and serious overdose cautions. Please see FDA MedlinePlus web site referenced at the end of this booklet for more information.

Withdrawals: If you stop taking this medication suddenly, you may experience withdrawal symptoms such as:

Anxiety
Chills
Cramps
Depression
Diarrhea
Difficulty falling asleep
Difficulty staying asleep
Fast breathing
Fast heartbeat
Irritability
Joint aches or pains
Loss of appetite
Muscle aches or pains

Nausea
Restlessness
Runny nose
Sneezing
Sweating
Vomiting
Watery eyes
Weakness
Yawning

Call your doctor if you have any withdrawal symptoms when your dose is decreased or when you stop taking oxycodone.

Important Warnings:

You should know that this medication may make you drowsy. Do not drive a car, operate heavy machinery, or participate in any other possibly dangerous activities until you know how this medication affects you.

Oxycodone may cause dizziness, lightheadedness, and fainting when you get up too quickly from a lying position.

See label or MedlinePlus web site for the full list of side effects and other warnings.

Brand Name: Percodan
Generic Name: oxycodone and aspirin

Type or Class of Drug: Opiate (narcotic) pain killer
A narcotic is a substance that dulls pain and induces sleep. Opiate means that is derived from or acts like opium in dulling the senses and inducing sleep.

Approved for: Relief of moderate to severe pain

Dependency and Addiction: Oxycodone can be habit-forming. Do not take a larger dose, take it more often, or take it for a longer period of time than prescribed by your doctor. If you have been taking oxycodone for more than a few days, do not stop taking oxycodone suddenly.

Oxycodone can produce drug dependence of the morphine type and, therefore, has the potential for being abused.

The aspirin part of this drug is not habit forming however it does have side effects and serious overdose cautions. Please see FDA MedlinePlus web site referenced at the end of this booklet for more information.

Withdrawals: If you stop taking this medication suddenly, you may experience withdrawal symptoms such as:

Anxiety
Chills
Cramps
Depression
Diarrhea
Difficulty falling asleep
Difficulty staying asleep
Fast breathing
Fast heartbeat
Irritability
Joint aches or pains
Loss of appetite
Muscle aches or pains
Nausea
Restlessness
Runny nose
Sneezing
Sweating
Vomiting
Watery eyes
Weakness
Yawning

Call your doctor if you have any withdrawal symptoms when your dose is decreased or when you stop taking oxycodone.

Important Warnings:

You should know that this medication may make you drowsy. Do not drive a car, operate heavy machinery, or participate in any other possibly dangerous activities until you know how this medication affects you.

Oxycodone may cause dizziness, lightheadedness, and fainting when you get up too quickly from a lying position.

See label or MedlinePlus web site for the full list of side effects and other warnings.

Brand Name: Pristiq
Generic Name: desvenlafaxine

Type or Class of Drug: Antidepressant

Approved for: Depression

Dependency and Addiction: Do not stop taking desvenlafaxine without talking to your doctor. Your doctor will probably decrease your dose gradually.

Withdrawals: If you suddenly stop taking desvenlafaxine, you may experience withdrawal symptoms such as:

Anxiety
Diarrhea
Difficulty falling asleep
Difficulty staying asleep
Dizziness
Extreme tiredness
Headache

Irritability
Nausea
Sweating
Unusual dreams

Tell your doctor if you experience any of these symptoms while you are decreasing your dose of desvenlafaxine or soon after you stop taking desvenlafaxine.

Important Warnings:

The Black Box Label placed by the FDA on antidepressants including Pristiq includes an extensive list of serious, life-threatening potential consequences. There is a tendency among medical professionals and of course with the pharmaceutical and psychiatric industry to downplay these warnings. Don't be fooled. These are real. They do happen and have happened to real people. The FDA does not place warnings like these lightly.

This Black Box Label includes the following warnings. Note that this is not the complete Black Box Label. That can be found at the FDA MedlinePlus website listed in the resources section at the end of this booklet.

* Children, teenagers, and young adults who take antidepressants to treat depression or other mental illnesses may be more likely to become suicidal than children, teenagers, and young adults who do not take antidepressants to treat these conditions.

* You should know that your mental health may change in unexpected ways when you take citalopram or other antidepressants even if you are an adult over 24 years of age. You may become suicidal, especially at the beginning of your treatment and any time that your dose is increased or decreased.

* You, your family, or your caregiver should call your doctor right away if you experience any of the following symptoms: Make sure someone around you such as a family member or friend or caregiver knows these symptoms so they can call the doctor if you are unable to seek treatment on your own.

Acting without thinking
Aggressive behavior
Agitation (suddenly violent and forceful, emotionally disturbed state of mind)
Difficulty falling asleep
Difficulty staying asleep
Extreme worry
Frenxied abnormal excitement
Irritability
New or worsening depression
Panic attacks
Planning to kill yourself
Severe restlessness
Thinking about harming yourself
Thinking about killing yourself
Trying to kill yourself

May make you drowsy and affect your judgment and thinking.

Brand Name: Provigil
Generic Name: modafinil

Type or Class of Drug: Wakefulness promoting agent

Approved for: Treatment of narcolepsy (a condition that causes excessive daytime sleepiness). Sometimes used for other sleep problems.

Dependency and Addiction: Modafinil may be habit-forming. Do not take a larger dose, take it more often, or take it for a longer period of time than prescribed by your doctor.

This drug can lead to dependence and has been known to be abused.

Withdrawals:

No specific withdrawals were observed during a trial however sleepiness returned in narcoleptic patients.

Feeling the need to continue taking the drug (addiction).

Important Warnings:

Modafinil should not be used in place of getting enough sleep
You should know that modafinil may affect your judgment or thinking.
Provigil (modafinil) may not completely relieve the sleepiness caused by your disorder
Do not drive a car or operate machinery until you know how this medication affects you.
Provigil cannot cure sleep disorders and it may not stop all of your sleepiness.

Brand Name: Prozac
Generic Name: fluoxetine

Type or Class of Drug: Antidepressant

Approved for: Depression, PMS, eating disorders, panic. OCD. Fluoxetine is also sometimes used to treat alcoholism, attention-deficit disorder, borderline personality disorder, sleep disorders, headaches, mental illness, posttraumatic stress disorder, Tourette's syndrome, obesity, sexual problems, and phobias.

Dependency and Addiction: Do not stop taking without talking to your doctor.

Withdrawals: If you suddenly stop taking fluoxetine, you may experience withdrawal symptoms such as:

Agitiation
Confusion
Dizziness
Difficulty falling asleep
Difficulty staying asleep
Dizziness
Headache
Irritability
Mood changes
Numbness
Tingling in the hands or feet
Tiredness

Important Warnings:

The Black Box Label placed by the FDA on antidepressants including Prozac includes an extensive list of serious, life-threatening potential consequences. There is a tendency among medical professionals and of course with the pharmaceutical and psychiatric industry to downplay these warnings. Don't be fooled. These are real. They do happen and have happened to real people. The FDA does not place warnings like these lightly.

This Black Box Label includes the following warnings. Note that this is not the complete Black Box Label. That can be found at the FDA MedlinePlus website listed in the resources section at the end of this booklet.

* Children, teenagers, and young adults who take antidepressants to treat depression or other mental illnesses may be more likely to become suicidal than children, teenagers, and young adults who do not take antidepressants to treat these conditions.

* You should know that your mental health may change in unexpected ways when you take Prozac or other antidepressants even if you are an adult over 24 years of age. You may become suicidal, especially at the beginning of your treatment and any time that your dose is increased or decreased.

* You, your family, or your caregiver should call your doctor right away if you experience any of the following symptoms: Make sure someone around you such as a family member or friend or caregiver knows these symptoms so they can call the doctor if you are unable to seek treatment on your own.

Acting without thinking
Aggressive behavior
Agitation (suddenly violent and forceful, emotionally disturbed state of mind)
Difficulty falling asleep
Difficulty staying asleep
Extreme worry
Frenxied abnormal excitement
Irritability
New or worsening depression
Panic attacks
Planning to kill yourself
Severe restlessness
Thinking about harming yourself
Thinking about killing yourself
Trying to kill yourself

May make you drowsy and affect your judgment and thinking.

Brand Name: Restoril
Generic Name: temazepam

Type or Class of Drug: Benzodiazepine - minor sedative
(One of the types of drugs used as tranquilizers or sedatives or
hypnotics or muscle relaxants; chronic use can lead to dependency)

Approved for: Used on a short-term basis to treat insomnia
(difficulty falling asleep or staying asleep).

Dependency and Addiction: Talk to your doctor before you stop
taking this medication. Your doctor will probably decrease your
dose gradually. Impaired control over drug use, compulsive use,
continued use despite harm, and craving

Withdrawals: If you suddenly stop taking temazepam, you may
experience the following:

Depression
Difficulty falling asleep
Difficulty staying asleep
Muscle cramps
Seizures (rarely)
Stomach cramps
Sweating
Uncontrollable shaking of a part of the body
Vomiting

Important Warnings:

Tell your doctor right away if you experience any of the following
symptoms:

Aggressive
Confusion
Difficulty concentrating
Feeling as if you are outside of your body

Hallucinations (seeing things or hearing voices that do not exist)
Memory problems
New depression
Other changes in your usual thoughts, mood or behavior
Strange or unusually outgoing behavior
Suicidal thoughts
Thinking about killing yourself
Worsening depression

Be sure that your family knows these symptoms so that they can call the doctor if you are unable to seek treatment on your own.

Brand Name: Risperdal
Generic Name: risperidone

Type or Class of Drug: Antipsychotic

Approved for: Schizophrenia (a mental illness that causes disturbed or unusual thinking, loss of interest in life, and strong or inappropriate emotions) in adults and teenagers 13 years of age and older. It is also used to treat episodes of mania (frenzied, abnormally excited, or irritated mood) or mixed episodes (symptoms of mania and depression that happen together) in adults and in teenagers and children 10 years of age and older with bipolar disorder (manic depressive disorder; a disease that causes episodes of depression, episodes of mania, and other abnormal moods). Risperidone is also used to treat behavior problems such as aggression, self-injury, and sudden mood changes in teenagers and children 5-16 years of age who have autism (a condition that causes repetitive behavior, difficulty interacting with others, and problems with communication).

Dependency and Addiction: Do not stop taking risperidone without talking to your doctor. If you suddenly stop taking risperidone, your symptoms may return and your illness may become harder to treat.

Withdrawals:

Delusions
Depression
Hallucinations
Insomnia
Irritability

Important Warnings:

The risk of developing tardive dyskinesia and the likelihood that it will become irreversible are believed to increase as the duration of treatment and the total cumulative dose of antipsychotic drugs administered to the patient increase. However, the syndrome can develop, although much less commonly, after relatively brief treatment periods at low doses.

Brand Name: Ritalin
Generic Name: methylphenidate

Type or Class of Drug: Central Nervous System Stimulant
[A stimulant is a drug that increases heart rate, breathing rate, brain function. And nervous system.]

Approved for: ADHD and Narcolepsy

Dependency and Addiction: Methylphenidate can be habit-forming. Methylphenidate can be habit-forming. Do not take a larger dose, take it more often, take it for a longer time, or take it in a different way than prescribed by your doctor. If you take too much methylphenidate, you may find that the medication no longer controls your symptoms, you may feel a need to take large amounts of the medication, and you may experience unusual changes in your behavior

Withdrawals:

Do not stop taking methylphenidate without talking to your doctor. The main withdrawal symptoms noted are:

Severe depression
Extreme fatigue
Changes in heart rhythm.

Important Warnings:

Methylphenidate may cause sudden death in children and teenagers, especially children or teenagers with heart defects or serious heart problems.

This medication also may cause sudden death, heart attack or stroke in adults, especially adults with heart defects or serious heart problems.

Methylphenidate may slow children's growth or weight gain.

Stimulants such as Concerta create a rise in blood pressure.

Stimulants may make any problems with behavior or problems a person is having with their thoughts worse than they were before taking the medication.

Aggressive behavior or hostility has been seen in connection with the taking of stimulants. This behavior should be watched for in patients taking Concerta.

Psychotic and manic symptoms such as hallucinations or delusional thinking can be caused by this drug in patients who have had not previous history of these feelings and problems. This can occur at just normal doses prescribed by a doctor.

Difficulty focusing and blurring of vision have been reported in people taking stimulant drugs such as Concerta.

There is some evidence stimulants may cause seizures.

Other adverse reactions to stimulants include:

Anxiety
Blood pressure increased
Decreased appetite
Dizziness
Dry mouth
Headache
Hyperhidrosis (excessive sweating)
Insomnia
Irritability
Nausea
Upper abdominal pain
Weight decreased

Brand Name: Roxanol
Generic Name: Morphine

Type or Class of Drug: Opiate (narcotic) pain reliever
A narcotic is a substance that dulls pain and induces sleep. Opiate means that is derived from or acts like opium in dulling the senses and inducing sleep.

Approved for: Treating moderate to severe pain

Dependency and Addiction: Morphine can be habit-forming. Take morphine exactly as directed. Do not take a larger dose, take it more often, or take it for a longer period of time or in a different way than prescribed by your doctor.
Physical dependence and tolerance are not unusual.

Withdrawals: Should not be abruptly discontinued. Do not stop taking morphine without talking to your doctor. Your doctor may decrease your dose gradually. If you suddenly stop taking morphine, you may experience withdrawal symptoms such as:

Abdominal cramps
Anorexia (loss of appetite especially as result of disease)
Anxiety
Backache
Chills
Coughing
Diarrhea
Difficulty falling asleep
Difficulty staying asleep
Hair on your skin standing on end
Hallucinating (seeing things or hearing voices that do not exist)
Increased blood pressure
Increased heart rate
Increased respiratory rate
Insomnia
Irritability
Joint pain
Myalgia (muscular pain or tenderness)
Mydriasis (prolonged and abnormal dilation (expanding, getting larger) of the pupil often due to drugs)
Nausea
Perspiration
Restlessness
Runny nose
Shaking of a part of your body that you cannot control
Sneezing
Sweating
Vomiting
Watery eyes
Weakness
Yawning

Important Warnings:

Morphine may cause dizziness, lightheadedness, and fainting when you get up too quickly from a lying position.

Ingestion of these capsules or of the pellets within the capsules may cause fatal respiratory depression when administered to patients not already tolerant to high doses of opioids.

Brand Name: Sarafem
Generic Name: fluoxetine

Type or Class of Drug: Antidepressant

Approved for: Depression: PMS, eating disorders, panic. OCD.
Fluoxetine is also sometimes used to treat alcoholism, attention-
deficit disorder, borderline personality disorder, sleep disorders,
headaches, mental illness, posttraumatic stress disorder, Tourette's
syndrome, obesity, sexual problems, and phobias.

Dependency and Addiction: Do not stop taking without talking to
your doctor.

Withdrawals: If you suddenly stop taking fluoxetine, you may
experience withdrawal symptoms such as:

Agitiation
Confusion
Dizziness
Difficulty falling asleep
Difficulty staying asleep
Dizziness
Headache
Irritability
Mood changes
Numbness
Tingling in the hands or feet
Tiredness

Important Warnings:

The Black Box Label placed by the FDA on antidepressants
including Pristiq includes an extensive list of serious, life-
threatening potential consequences. There is a tendency among
medical professionals and of course with the pharmaceutical and
psychiatric industry to downplay these warnings. Don't be fooled.
These are real. They do happen and have happened to real people.
The FDA does not place warnings like these lightly.

This Black Box Label includes the following warnings. Note that this is not the complete Black Box Label. That can be found at the FDA MedlinePlus website listed in the resources section at the end of this booklet.

* Children, teenagers, and young adults who take antidepressants to treat depression or other mental illnesses may be more likely to become suicidal than children, teenagers, and young adults who do not take antidepressants to treat these conditions.

* You should know that your mental health may change in unexpected ways when you take citalopram or other antidepressants even if you are an adult over 24 years of age. You may become suicidal, especially at the beginning of your treatment and any time that your dose is increased or decreased.

* You, your family, or your caregiver should call your doctor right away if you experience any of the following symptoms: Make sure someone around you such as a family member or friend or caregiver knows these symptoms so they can call the doctor if you are unable to seek treatment on your own.

Acting without thinking
Aggressive behavior
Agitation (suddenly violent and forceful, emotionally disturbed state of mind)
Difficulty falling asleep
Difficulty staying asleep
Extreme worry
Frenxied abnormal excitement
Irritability
New or worsening depression
Panic attacks
Planning to kill yourself
Severe restlessness
Thinking about harming yourself
Thinking about killing yourself
Trying to kill yourself

May make you drowsy and affect your judgment and thinking.

Brand Name: Seconal
Generic Name: secobarbital

Type or Class of Drug: Barbiturate

Approved for: Used on a short-term basis to treat insomnia (difficulty falling asleep or staying asleep), also used to treat anxiety before surgery

Dependency and Addiction: Do not stop taking secobarbital without talking to your doctor. Your doctor will probably decrease your dose gradually.

Secobarbital should normally be taken for short periods of time. If you take secobarbital for 2 weeks or longer, secobarbital may not help you sleep as well as it did when you first began to take the medication. If you take secobarbital for a long time, you may also develop dependence ('addiction,' a need to continue taking the medication) on secobarbital.

Talk to your doctor about the risks of taking secobarbital for 2 weeks or longer. Do not take a larger dose of secobarbital, take it more often, or take it for a longer time than prescribed by your doctor.

Withdrawals: If you suddenly stop taking secobarbital, you may develop:

Anxiety
Changes in vision
Difficulty falling asleep
Difficulty staying asleep
Dizziness
Muscle twitching
Nausea
Uncontrollable shaking of your hands or fingers
Vomiting
Weakness

Or you may experience more severe withdrawal symptoms such as seizures or extreme confusion.

Important Warnings:

You should know that some people who took medications for sleep got out of bed and drove their cars, prepared and ate food, had sex, made phone calls, or were involved in other activities while partially asleep. After they woke up, these people were usually unable to remember what they had done.

Call your doctor right away if you find out that you have been driving or doing anything else while you were sleeping.

You should know that this medication may make you drowsy during the daytime. Do not drive a car or operate machinery until you know how this medication affects you.

Brand Name: Seroquel
Generic Name: quetiapine

Type or Class of Drug: Antipsychotic

Approved for: Treatment of Schizophrenia (a mental illness that causes disturbed or unusual thinking, loss of interest in life, and strong or inappropriate emotions).
Also used to treat mania, depression, bipolar disorder and to treat schizophrenia and bipolar disorder in children. (However see the FDA's Black Label Warning before allowing this to be given to your child)
Dependency and Addiction: Do not stop taking quetiapine without talking to your doctor. Your doctor will probably want to decrease your dose gradually.

Withdrawals: If you suddenly stop taking quetiapine, you may experience withdrawal symptoms such as:

Diarrhea
Difficulty falling asleep
Difficulty staying asleep
Dizziness
Headache
Insomnia
Irritability
Nausea
Vomiting

Important Warnings: The Black Box Label placed by the FDA on antidepressants including quetiapine includes an extensive list of serious, life-threatening potential consequences. There is a tendency among medical professionals and of course with the pharmaceutical and psychiatric industry to downplay these warnings. Don't be fooled. These are real. They do happen and have happened to real people. The FDA does not place warnings like these lightly.

This Black Box Label includes the following warnings. Note that this is not the complete Black Box Label. That can be found at the FDA MedlinePlus website listed in the resources section at the end of this booklet.

* Children, teenagers, and young adults who take antidepressants to treat depression or other mental illnesses may be more likely to become suicidal than children, teenagers, and young adults who do not take antidepressants to treat these conditions.

* You should know that your mental health may change in unexpected ways when you take quetiapine or other antidepressants even if you are an adult over 24 years of age. You may become suicidal, especially at the beginning of your treatment and any time that your dose is increased or decreased.

* You, your family, or your caregiver should call your doctor right away if you experience any of the following symptoms: Make sure someone around you such as a family member or friend or caregiver knows these symptoms so they can call the doctor if you are unable to seek treatment on your own.

Acting without thinking
Aggressive behavior
Agitation (suddenly violent and forceful, emotionally disturbed state of mind)
Difficulty falling asleep
Difficulty staying asleep
Extreme worry
Frenxied abnormal excitement
Irritability
New or worsening depression
Panic attacks
Planning to kill yourself
Severe restlessness
Thinking about harming yourself
Thinking about killing yourself
Trying to kill yourself

The risk of developing tardive dyskinesia and the likelihood that it will become irreversible are believed to increase as the duration of treatment and the total cumulative dose of antipsychotic drugs administered to the patient increase. However, the syndrome can develop, although much less commonly, after relatively brief treatment periods at low doses or may even arise after discontinuation of treatment.

Studies have shown that older adults with dementia (a brain disorder that affects the ability to remember, think clearly, communicate, and perform daily activities and that may cause changes in mood and personality) who take antipsychotics (medications for mental illness) such as quetiapine have an increased risk of death during treatment.

You should know that quetiapine may make it harder for your body to cool down when it gets very hot.

Brand Name: Soma
Generic Name: carisoprodol

Type or Class of Drug: Muscle relaxant

Approved for: Used with rest, physical therapy, and other measures to relax muscles and relieve pain and discomfort caused by strains, sprains, and other muscle injuries.

Dependency and Addiction: Withdrawal, and abuse have been reported with prolonged use. Do not stop using Soma suddenly without first talking to your doctor. You may need to use less and less before you stop the medication completely.

Withdrawals:

Convulsions
Dependence
Headache
Nausea
Pain
Seizures
Sleep problems

Important Warnings:

Soma should only be used for short periods (up to two or three weeks) because adequate evidence of effectiveness for more prolonged use has not been established.

Do not stop using Soma suddenly without first talking to your doctor. You may need to use less and less before you stop the medication completely.

Brand Name: Sonata
Generic Name: zaleplon

Type or Class of Drug: Hypnotic

Approved for: Used to treat insomnia (difficulty falling asleep

Dependency and Addiction: Do not stop taking Sonata without first talking to your doctor.

Withdrawals: If you suddenly stop taking zaleplon, you may experience withdrawal symptoms such as:

Muscle cramps
Seizures
Shakiness
Stomach cramps
Sweating
Unpleasant feelings
Vomiting

Important Warnings:

You should know that your mental health may change in unexpected ways while you are taking this medication.

Tell your doctor right away if you experience any of the following symptoms:

Aggressiveness
Any other changes in your usual thoughts or behavior
Confusion
Feeling as if you are outside of your body
Hallucinations (seeing things or hearing voices that do not exist)
Memory problems
New depression
Strange or unusually outgoing behavior
Thinking about killing yourself
Worsening depression

Be sure that your family knows these symptoms so that they can call the doctor if you are unable to seek treatment on your own.

Brand Name: Thorazine
Generic Name: chlorpromazine

Type or Class of Drug: Antipsychotic, major tranquilizer

Approved for: Chlorpromazine is used to treat the symptoms of schizophrenia (a mental illness that causes disturbed or unusual thinking, loss of interest in life, and strong or inappropriate emotions) and other psychotic disorders (conditions that cause difficulty telling the difference between things or ideas that are real and things or ideas that are not real) and to treat the symptoms of mania (frenzied, abnormally excited mood) in people who have bipolar disorder (manic depressive disorder; a condition that causes episodes of mania, episodes of depression, and other abnormal moods).

Chlorpromazine is also used to treat severe behavior problems such as explosive, aggressive behavior and hyperactivity in children 1-12 years of age. Chlorpromazine is also used to control nausea and vomiting, to relieve hiccups that have lasted one month or longer, and to relieve restlessness and nervousness that may occur just before surgery.

Dependency and Addiction: Do not stop taking chlorpromazine without talking to your doctor. Your doctor will probably decrease your dose gradually.

Withdrawals: If you suddenly stop taking chlorpromazine, you may experience withdrawal symptoms, such as:

Dizziness
Gastritis
Nausea
Shakiness
Stomach pain
Tremulousness
Vomiting

Important Warnings:

Both the risk of developing tardive dyskinesia and the likelihood that it will become irreversible are believed to increase as the duration of treatment and the total cumulative dose of antipsychotic drugs administered to the patient increase. However, the syndrome can develop, although much less commonly, after relatively brief treatment periods at low doses.

Studies have shown that older adults with dementia (a brain disorder that affects the ability to remember, think clearly, communicate, and perform daily activities and that may cause changes in mood and personality) who take antipsychotics (medications for mental illness) such as chlorpromazine have an increased chance of death during treatment.

You should know that chlorpromazine may cause dizziness, lightheadedness, fast heartbeat, and fainting, especially when you get up too quickly from a lying position.

Brand Name: Tylox
Generic Name: acetaminophen and oxycodone

Type or Class of Drug: Opiate (narcotic) pain killer
A narcotic is a substance that dulls pain and induces sleep. Opiate means that is derived from or acts like opium in dulling the senses and inducing sleep.

Approved for: To relieve moderate to severe pain

Dependency and Addiction: Oxycodone can be habit-forming. Do not take a larger dose, take it more often, or take it for a longer period of time than prescribed by your doctor. If you have been taking oxycodone for more than a few days, do not stop taking oxycodone suddenly.

Oxycodone can produce drug dependence of the morphine type and, therefore, has the potential for being abused.

The acetaminophen part of this drug is not habit forming however it does have side effects and serious overdose cautions. Please see FDA MedlinePlus web site referenced at the end of this booklet for more information.

Withdrawals: If you stop taking this medication suddenly, you may experience withdrawal symptoms such as:

Anxiety
Chills
Cramps
Depression
Diarrhea
Difficulty falling asleep
Difficulty staying asleep
Fast breathing
Fast heartbeat
Irritability
Joint aches or pains
Loss of appetite
Muscle aches or pains
Nausea
Restlessness
Runny nose
Sneezing
Sweating
Vomiting
Watery eyes
Weakness
Yawning

Call your doctor if you have any withdrawal symptoms when your dose is decreased or when you stop taking oxycodone.

Important Warnings:

You should know that this medication may make you drowsy. Do not drive a car, operate heavy machinery, or participate in any other possibly dangerous activities until you know how this medication affects you.

Oxycodone may cause dizziness, lightheadedness, and fainting when you get up too quickly from a lying position.

See label or MedlinePlus web site for the full list of side effects and other warnings.

Brand Name: Valium
Generic Name: diazepam

Type or Class of Drug: Benzodiazepine - minor sedative
(One of the types of drugs used as tranquilizers or sedatives or hypnotics or muscle relaxants; chronic use can lead to dependency)

Approved for: Used to relieve anxiety, muscle spasms, and seizures and to control agitation caused by alcohol withdrawal.

Diazepam is also used to treat irritable bowel syndrome and panic attacks

Dependency and Addiction: Diazepam can be habit-forming. Do not take a larger dose, take it more often, or for a longer time than your doctor tells you to. Tolerance may develop with long-term or excessive use, making the drug less effective. This medication must be taken regularly to be effective. Do not skip doses even if you feel that you do not need them. Do not take diazepam for more than 4 months or stop taking this medication without talking to your doctor.

Stopping the drug suddenly can worsen your condition.

Withdrawals: Stopping the drug suddenly can cause withdrawals such as:

Abdominal cramps
Anxiousness
Convulsions
Irritability
Muscle cramps
Sleeplessness
Sweating
Tremor
Vomiting

Important Warnings:

To assure the safe and effective use of benzodiazepines, patients should be informed that, since benzodiazepines may produce psychological and physical dependence.

Paradoxical reactions such as the following have been reported:

Anxiety
Hallucinations
Insomnia
Muscle tone increased with an exaggeration of tendon reflexes
Rage
Sleep disturbances
Stimulation
Unusual or excessive excitement

Should these occur, use of this drug should be discontinued.

Please take a good look at all the side effects listed here:
www.nlm.nih.gov/medlineplus/druginfo/meds/a682047.html#brand-name-1

Brand Name: Vicodin
Generic Name: Hydrocodone and acetaminophen

Type or Class of Drug: Opiate (narcotic) pain killer
A narcotic is a substance that dulls pain and induces sleep. Opiate means that is derived from or acts like opium in dulling the senses and inducing sleep.

Approved for: Treatment of moderate to severe pain and coughing

Dependency and Addiction: Hydrocodone may be habit-forming. Take hydrocodone exactly as directed. Do not take a larger dose, take it more often, or take it for a longer period of time than prescribed by your doctor. Call your doctor if you develop a strong desire to take more medication than prescribed.

The acetaminophen part of this drug is not habit forming however it does have side effects and serious overdose cautions. Please see FDA MedlinePlus web site referenced at the end of this booklet for more information.

Withdrawals: If you suddenly stop taking hydrocodone, you may experience withdrawal symptoms.

Anxiety
Back pain
Chills
Cravings
Depression
Diarrhea
Fatigue
Feeling sick
Flu-like symptoms
Insomnia
Irritability
Loss of appetite
Muscle aches
Muscle pains
Runny nose
Sleep disturbances
Sweating

Watery eyes
Yawning

Important Warnings:

"Doctor shopping" to obtain additional prescriptions is common among drug abusers and people suffering from untreated addiction.

Call your doctor if your symptoms are not controlled by the hydrocodone product you are taking. Do not increase your dose of medication on your own.

Hydrocodone may make you drowsy. Do not drive a car or operate machinery until you know how this medication affects you.

Brand Name: Vyvance
Generic Name: lisdexamfetamine

Type or Class of Drug: Central Nervous System Stimulant

Approved for: ADHD

Dependency and Addiction: Lisdexamfetamine can be habit-forming. Do not take a larger dose, take it more often, take it for a longer time, or take it in a different way than prescribed by your doctor. If you take too much lisdexamfetamine, you may find that the medication no longer controls your symptoms, you may feel a need to take large amounts of the medication, and you may experience symptoms such as rash, difficulty falling asleep or staying asleep, irritability, hyperactivity, and unusual changes in your personality or behavior.

Overusing lisdexamfetamine may also cause sudden death or serious heart problems, such as heart attack or stroke.

Withdrawals:

Your doctor will probably decrease your dose gradually and monitor you carefully during this time.

If you suddenly stop taking Vyvanse you may develop:
Extreme tiredness
Severe depression

Important Warnings:

Overusing lisdexamfetamine may also cause sudden death or serious heart problems, such as heart attack or stroke.

Chronic use and dependence may result in:

Hyperactivity (a condition characterized by excessive restlessness and movement)
Insomnia
Irritability
Personality changes
Psychosis
Schizophrenia
Skin disease

You should know that this medication may make it difficult for you to perform activities that require alertness or physical coordination. Do not drive a car or operate machinery until you know how this medication affects you.

Brand Name: Wellbutrin / Wellbutrin XR
Generic Name: bupropion

Type or Class of Drug: Antidepressant

Approved for: Depression and as Zyban, bupropion is approved for smoking cessation

Dependency and Addiction: Do not stop taking bupropion without talking to your doctor. Your doctor will probably decrease your dose gradually.

Withdrawals:

Agitation (suddenly violent and forceful, emotionally disturbed state of mind)
Anxiety
Burning sensation
Confusion
Dizziness
Headaches
Insomnia
Irritability
Tingling sensation
Tiredness

Important Warnings:

The Black Box Label placed by the FDA on antidepressants including bupropion includes an extensive list of serious, life-threatening potential consequences. There is a tendency among medical professionals and of course with the pharmaceutical and psychiatric industry to downplay these warnings. Don't be fooled. These are real. They do happen and have happened to real people. The FDA does not place warnings like these lightly.

This Black Box Label includes the following warnings. Note that this is not the complete Black Box Label. That can be found at the FDA MedlinePlus website listed in the resources section at the end of this booklet.

* Children, teenagers, and young adults who take antidepressants to treat depression or other mental illnesses may be more likely to become suicidal than children, teenagers, and young adults who do not take antidepressants to treat these conditions.

* You should know that your mental health may change in unexpected ways when you take bupropion or other antidepressants even if you are an adult over 24 years of age. You may become suicidal, especially at the beginning of your treatment and any time that your dose is increased or decreased.

* You, your family, or your caregiver should call your doctor right away if you experience any of the following symptoms: Make sure someone around you such as a family member or friend or caregiver knows these symptoms so they can call the doctor if you are unable to seek treatment on your own.

Acting without thinking
Aggressive behavior
Agitation (suddenly violent and forceful, emotionally disturbed state of mind)
Difficulty falling asleep
Difficulty staying asleep
Extreme worry
Frenxied abnormal excitement
Irritability
New or worsening depression
Panic attacks
Planning to kill yourself
Severe restlessness
Thinking about harming yourself
Thinking about killing yourself
Trying to kill yourself

Serious neuropsychiatric events, including but not limited to depression, suicidal ideation, suicide attempt, and completed suicide have been reported in patients taking bupropion for smoking cessation.

All patients being treated with bupropion for smoking cessation treatment should be observed for neuropsychiatric symptoms including changes in behavior, hostility, agitation, depressed mood, and suicide-related events, including ideation, behavior, and attempted suicide.

If you experience any of the following symptoms, stop taking bupropion and call your doctor immediately (make sure a friend or family member is aware of these potential effects so they can contact your doctor or emergency if you are unable to do so or are unaware of any of these changes in yourself):

Abnormal sensations
Abnormal thoughts
Agitation (suddenly violent and forceful, emotionally disturbed state of mind)
Angry behavior
Any other sudden or unusual changes in behavior
Anxiety
Dangerous behavior
Feeling confused
Feeling that people are against your
Hallucinations (seeing things or hearing voices that do not exist)
Mania (frenzied, abnormally excited or irritated mood);
New depression
Panic attacks
Restlessness
Suicidal actions
Suicidal thoughts
Violent behavior
Worsening depression

Brand Name: Xanax
Generic Name: alprazolam

Type or Class of Drug: Benzodiazepine - minor sedative
(One of the types of drugs used as tranquilizers or sedatives or
hypnotics or muscle relaxants; chronic use can lead to dependency)

Approved for: Treatment of Anxiety and Panic,   Sometimes to
treat depression, fear of open spaces (agoraphobia), and
premenstrual syndrome

Dependency and Addiction: Certain adverse clinical events, some
life-threatening, are a direct consequence of physical dependence to
Xanax. Xanax can be habit-forming. Do not take a larger dose or
take it more often or for a longer time than your doctor tells you to.
Do not stop taking alprazolam without talking to your doctor. Your
doctor will decrease your dose gradually.

Withdrawals: Suddenly stopping to take alprazolam may worsen
your condition and cause withdrawal symptoms. Withdrawal
symptoms include:

Anxiousness
Anxiety
Appetite decrease
Blurred vision
Diarrhea
Dysosmia
Heightened sensory perception
Impaired concentration
Inability to think clearly and concentrate
Insomnia
Irritability
Muscle cramps
Muscle twitch
Seizures
Sleeplessness
Tingling and numbness
Weight loss

Important Warnings:

Some life-threatening adverse events are a direct consequence of physical dependence on Xanax.

Some side effects can be serious. The following symptoms are uncommon, but if you experience any of them, call your doctor immediately:

Confusion
Memory problems
Problems with coordination
Seeing things or hearing voices that do not exist
Seizures
Severe skin rash
Yellowing of the skin eyes

Brand Name: Zoloft
Generic Name: sertraline

Type or Class of Drug: Antidepressant

Approved for: Sertraline is used to treat depression, obsessive-compulsive disorder (bothersome thoughts that won't go away and the need to perform certain actions over and over), panic attacks (sudden, unexpected attacks of extreme fear and worry about these attacks), posttraumatic stress disorder (disturbing psychological symptoms that develop after a frightening experience), and social anxiety disorder (extreme fear of interacting with others or performing in front of others that interferes with normal life). It is also used to relieve the symptoms of premenstrual dysphoric disorder, including mood swings, irritability, bloating, and breast tenderness. Sertraline is also used sometimes to treat headaches and sexual problems.

Dependency and Addiction: Do not stop taking sertraline without talking to your doctor.

Withdrawals:

Abdominal pain
Agitation (suddenly violent and forceful, emotionally disturbed state of mind)
Anxiety
Diarrhea
Dizziness
Dry Mouth
Dyspepsia
Ejaculation failure
Fatigue
Headache
Hot flush
Insomnia
Nausea
Nervousness
Palpitations
Somnolence
Tremors

Important Warnings:

The Black Box Label placed by the FDA on antidepressants including bupropion includes an extensive list of serious, life-threatening potential consequences. There is a tendency among medical professionals and of course with the pharmaceutical and psychiatric industry to downplay these warnings. Don't be fooled. These are real. They do happen and have happened to real people. The FDA does not place warnings like these lightly.

This Black Box Label includes the following warnings. Note that this is not the complete Black Box Label. That can be found at the FDA MedlinePlus website listed in the resources section at the end of this booklet.

* Children, teenagers, and young adults who take antidepressants to treat depression or other mental illnesses may be more likely to become suicidal than children, teenagers, and young adults who do not take antidepressants to treat these conditions.

* You should know that your mental health may change in unexpected ways when you take bupropion or other antidepressants even if you are an adult over 24 years of age. You may become suicidal, especially at the beginning of your treatment and any time that your dose is increased or decreased.

* You, your family, or your caregiver should call your doctor right away if you experience any of the following symptoms: Make sure someone around you such as a family member or friend or caregiver knows these symptoms so they can call the doctor if you are unable to seek treatment on your own.

Acting without thinking
Aggressive behavior
Agitation (suddenly violent and forceful, emotionally disturbed state of mind)
Difficulty falling asleep
Difficulty staying asleep
Extreme worry
Frenxied abnormal excitement
Irritability
New or worsening depression
Panic attacks
Planning to kill yourself
Severe restlessness
Thinking about harming yourself
Thinking about killing yourself
Trying to kill yourself

Brand Name: Zyban
Generic Name: bupropion

Type or Class of Drug: Antidepressant

Approved for: Depression and as Zyban, bupropion is approved for smoking cessation

Dependency and Addiction: Do not stop taking bupropion without talking to your doctor. Your doctor will probably decrease your dose gradually.

Withdrawals:

Agitation (suddenly violent and forceful, emotionally disturbed state of mind)
Anxiety
Burning sensation
Confusion
Dizziness
Headaches
Insomnia
Irritability
Tingling sensation
Tiredness

Important Warnings:

The Black Box Label placed by the FDA on antidepressants including bupropion includes an extensive list of serious, life-threatening potential consequences. There is a tendency among medical professionals and of course with the pharmaceutical and psychiatric industry to downplay these warnings. Don't be fooled. These are real. They do happen and have happened to real people. The FDA does not place warnings like these lightly.

This Black Box Label includes the following warnings. Note that this is not the complete Black Box Label. That can be found at the FDA MedlinePlus website listed in the resources section at the end of this booklet.

* Children, teenagers, and young adults who take antidepressants to treat depression or other mental illnesses may be more likely to become suicidal than children, teenagers, and young adults who do not take antidepressants to treat these conditions.

* You should know that your mental health may change in unexpected ways when you take bupropion or other antidepressants even if you are an adult over 24 years of age. You may become suicidal, especially at the beginning of your treatment and any time that your dose is increased or decreased.

* You, your family, or your caregiver should call your doctor right away if you experience any of the following symptoms: Make sure someone around you such as a family member or friend or caregiver knows these symptoms so they can call the doctor if you are unable to seek treatment on your own.

Acting without thinking
Aggressive behavior
Agitation (suddenly violent and forceful, emotionally disturbed state of mind)
Difficulty falling asleep
Difficulty staying asleep
Extreme worry
Frenxied abnormal excitement
Irritability
New or worsening depression
Panic attacks
Planning to kill yourself
Severe restlessness
Thinking about harming yourself
Thinking about killing yourself
Trying to kill yourself

Serious neuropsychiatric events, including but not limited to depression, suicidal ideation, suicide attempt, and completed suicide have been reported in patients taking bupropion for smoking cessation.

All patients being treated with bupropion for smoking cessation treatment should be observed for neuropsychiatric symptoms including changes in behavior, hostility, agitation, depressed mood, and suicide-related events, including ideation, behavior, and attempted suicide.

If you experience any of the following symptoms, stop taking bupropion and call your doctor immediately (make sure a friend or family member is aware of these potential effects so they can contact your doctor or emergency if you are unable to do so or are unaware of any of these changes in yourself):

Abnormal sensations
Abnormal thoughts
Agitation (suddenly violent and forceful, emotionally disturbed state of mind)
Angry behavior
Any other sudden or unusual changes in behavior
Anxiety
Dangerous behavior
Feeling confused
Feeling that people are against your
Hallucinations (seeing things or hearing voices that do not exist)
Mania (frenzied, abnormally excited or irritated mood);
New depression
Panic attacks
Restlessness
Suicidal actions
Suicidal thoughts
Violent behavior
Worsening depression

Brand Name: Zyprexa
Generic Name: olanzapine

Type or Class of Drug: Antipsychotic

Approved for: To treat the symptoms of schizophrenia. It is also used to treat bipolar disorder

Dependency and Addiction: Do not stop taking olanzapine without talking to your doctor. Your doctor will probably want to decrease your dose gradually.

Withdrawals:

Zyprexa withdrawal symptoms can include, but are not limited to:

Being suspicious
Being withdrawn
Believing things that aren't true
Delusions
Depression
Hallucinations (seeing or hearing things that aren't there)
Hearing voices
Insomnia
Mania
Symptoms of schizophrenia

Important Warnings:

The risk of developing tardive dyskinesia and the likelihood that it will become irreversible are believed to increase as the duration of treatment and the total cumulative dose of antipsychotic drugs administered to the patient increase. However, the syndrome can develop, although much less commonly, after relatively brief treatment periods at low doses or may even arise after discontinuation of treatment.

Older adults with dementia may also have a greater chance of having a stroke or mini-stroke during treatment. If you experience any of the following symptoms, call your doctor immediately: slow or difficult speech, sudden dizziness or faintness, or weakness or numbness of an arm or leg.

You should know that olanzapine may cause fast or slow heartbeat, dizziness, lightheadedness, and fainting when you get up too quickly from a lying position.

Teenagers who take olanzapine are more likely than adults who take olanzapine to gain weight, have increased levels of fat in their blood, develop liver problems, and experience side effects such as sleepiness, breast enlargement, and discharge from the breasts.

Alphabetically by Generic Name

Generic Name: alprazolam
Brand Name: Xanax

Type or Class of Drug: Benzodiazepine - minor sedative
(One of the types of drugs used as tranquilizers or sedatives or
hypnotics or muscle relaxants; chronic use can lead to dependency)

Approved for: Treatment of Anxiety and Panic, Sometimes to
treat depression, fear of open spaces (agoraphobia), and
premenstrual syndrome

Dependency and Addiction: Certain adverse clinical events, some
life-threatening, are a direct consequence of physical dependence to
Xanax. Xanax can be habit-forming. Do not take a larger dose or
take it more often or for a longer time than your doctor tells you to.
Do not stop taking alprazolam without talking to your doctor. Your
doctor will decrease your dose gradually.

Withdrawals: Suddenly stopping to take alprazolam may worsen
your condition and cause withdrawal symptoms. Withdrawal
symptoms may be worse if you take more than 4 mg of alprazolam
every day. Withdrawal symptoms include:

Anxiousness
Anxiety
Appetite decrease
Blurred vision
Diarrhea
Dysosmia
Heightened sensory perception
Impaired concentration
Inability to think clearly and concentrate
Insomnia
Irritability
Muscle cramps
Muscle twitch
Seizures

Sleeplessness
Tingling and numbness
Weight loss

Important Warnings:

Some life-threatening adverse events are a direct consequence of physical dependence on Xanax.

Some side effects can be serious. The following symptoms are uncommon, but if you experience any of them, call your doctor immediately:

Confusion
Memory problems
Problems with coordination
Seeing things or hearing voices that do not exist
Seizures
Severe skin rash
Yellowing of the skin eyes

Generic Name: amphetamine / dextroamphetamine
Brand Name: Adderall / Adderall XR

Type or Class of Drug: Central Nervous System Stimulant
[A stimulant is a drug that increases heart rate, breathing rate, brain function. And nervous system.]

Approved for: Treatment of ADHD in adults and children and for treatment of narcolepsy (asleep disorder that causes excessive sleepiness during the daytime and sudden attacks of sleep)

Dependency and Addiction: Adderall and Adderall XR can be habit-forming. Amphetamines (one of the ingredients in Adderall) have a high potential for abuse. Taking amphetamines for a prolonged period may lead to drug dependence. The drugs should be prescribed and dispensed sparingly.

If you take too much dextroamphetamine and amphetamine, you may find that the medication no longer controls your symptoms

You may feel a need to take large amounts of the medication.

Amphetamines have been extensively abused. Tolerance, extreme dependence and severe social disability have occurred.

Withdrawals:

Abruptly stopping this drug after taking high doses can result in withdrawal symptoms including:

Depression
Extreme fatigue
Hyperactivity (a condition characterized by excessive restlessness and movement)
Insomnia
Irritability
Personality changes
Psychosis, often indistinguishable from schizophrenia (psychosis is defined as a loss of contact with reality where the person gets false ideas about what is taking place or who he is and has hallucinations, seeing or hearing things that aren'there)

Severe dermatoses (Skin problems)

Important Warnings: Adderall and Adderall XR have many warnings including the FDA's Black Box Warning. These warnings include:

Misuse of amphetamines may cause sudden death and serious cardiovascular adverse events (like heart attacks).

Dextroamphetamine and amphetamine may slow children's growth or weight gain.

You may experience symptoms such as rash, difficulty falling asleep or staying asleep, irritability, hyperactivity, and unusual changes in your personality or behavior.

Overusing Adderall or Adderall XR may also cause sudden death or serious heart problems such as heart attack or stroke.

Even if you or your child or loved one is taking exactly the amount prescribed, please be aware of the above important warnings and contact your doctor immediately if any of the above should occur.

Remember this drug is addictive and included in the effects of taking too much are changes in the patient's personality or behavior. So extra caution should be taken to contact a doctor the moment you sense any possible change.

Since this drug is often abused it's important to keep track of how many tablets or capsules are left so you will know if any are missing.

This medication also may cause sudden death, heart attack, or stroke in adults, especially adults with heart defects or serious heart problems.

Adderall and Adderall XR may cause sudden death in children and teenagers, especially children and teenagers who have heart defects or serious heart problems.

Generic Name: bupropion
Brand Name: Wellbutrin / Wellbutrin XR / Zyban

Type or Class of Drug: Antidepressant

Approved for: Depression and as Zyban, bupropion is approved for smoking cessation

Dependency and Addiction: Do not stop taking bupropion without talking to your doctor. Your doctor will probably decrease your dose gradually.

Withdrawals:

Agitation (suddenly violent and forceful, emotionally disturbed state of mind)
Anxiety
Burning sensation
Confusion
Dizziness
Headaches
Insomnia
Irritability
Tingling sensation
Tiredness

Important Warnings:

The Black Box Label placed by the FDA on antidepressants including bupropion includes an extensive list of serious, life-threatening potential consequences. There is a tendency among medical professionals and of course with the pharmaceutical and psychiatric industry to downplay these warnings. Don't be fooled. These are real. They do happen and have happened to real people. The FDA does not place warnings like these lightly.

This Black Box Label includes the following warnings. Note that this is not the complete Black Box Label. That can be found at the FDA MedlinePlus website listed in the resources section at the end of this booklet.

* Children, teenagers, and young adults who take antidepressants to treat depression or other mental illnesses may be more likely to become suicidal than children, teenagers, and young adults who do not take antidepressants to treat these conditions.

* You should know that your mental health may change in unexpected ways when you take bupropion or other antidepressants even if you are an adult over 24 years of age. You may become suicidal, especially at the beginning of your treatment and any time that your dose is increased or decreased.

* You, your family, or your caregiver should call your doctor right away if you experience any of the following symptoms: Make sure someone around you such as a family member or friend or caregiver knows these symptoms so they can call the doctor if you are unable to seek treatment on your own.

Acting without thinking
Aggressive behavior
Agitation (suddenly violent and forceful, emotionally disturbed state of mind)
Difficulty falling asleep
Difficulty staying asleep
Extreme worry
Frenxied abnormal excitement
Irritability
New or worsening depression
Panic attacks
Planning to kill yourself
Severe restlessness
Thinking about harming yourself
Thinking about killing yourself
Trying to kill yourself

Serious neuropsychiatric events, including but not limited to depression, suicidal ideation, suicide attempt, and completed suicide have been reported in patients taking bupropion for smoking cessation.

All patients being treated with bupropion for smoking cessation treatment should be observed for neuropsychiatric symptoms including changes in behavior, hostility, agitation, depressed mood, and suicide-related events, including ideation, behavior, and attempted suicide.

If you experience any of the following symptoms, stop taking bupropion and call your doctor immediately (make sure a friend or family member is aware of these potential effects so they can contact your doctor or emergency if you are unable to do so or are unaware of any of these changes in yourself):

Abnormal sensations
Abnormal thoughts
Agitation (suddenly violent and forceful, emotionally disturbed state of mind)
Angry behavior
Any other sudden or unusual changes in behavior
Anxiety
Dangerous behavior
Feeling confused
Feeling that people are against your
Hallucinations (seeing things or hearing voices that do not exist)
Mania (frenzied, abnormally excited or irritated mood);
New depression
Panic attacks
Restlessness
Suicidal actions
Suicidal thoughts
Violent behavior
Worsening depression

Generic Name: buspirone
Brand Name: Buspar

Type or Class of Drug: Anti-anxiety

Approved for: Short-term treatment for relief of anxiety.
Sometimes used for premenstrual symptoms.

Dependency and Addiction: Do not stop taking buspirone without
talking to your doctor, especially if you have taken large doses for a
long time. Your doctor probably will decrease your dose gradually.

Withdrawals:

Abdominal cramps
Agitation (suddenly violent and forceful, emotionally disturbed state
of mind)
Anxiety
Flu-like symptoms without fever
Insomnia
Irrtability
Muscle cramps
Seizures (occasionally)
Sweating
Vomiting

Important Warnings:

Patients should be cautioned about operating an automobile or using
heavy or complex machinery until they are reasonably certain that
buspirone does not affect them adversely.

The more commonly observed adverse events associated with the
use of BuSpar include
Dizziness
Excitement
Headache
Light-headedness
Nervousness

Generic Name: carisoprodol
Brand Name: Soma

Type or Class of Drug: Muscle relaxant

Approved for: Used with rest, physical therapy, and other measures to relax muscles and relieve pain and discomfort caused by strains, sprains, and other muscle injuries.

Dependency and Addiction: Withdrawal, and abuse have been reported with prolonged use. Do not stop using Soma suddenly without first talking to your doctor. You may need to use less and less before you stop the medication completely.

Withdrawals:

Convulsions
Dependence
Headache
Nausea
Pain
Seizures
Sleep problems

Important Warnings:

Soma should only be used for short periods (up to two or three weeks) because adequate evidence of effectiveness for more prolonged use has not been established.

Do not stop using Soma suddenly without first talking to your doctor. You may need to use less and less before you stop the medication completely.

Generic Name: chlordiazepoxide
Brand Name: Librium

Type or Class of Drug: Benzodiazepine - minor sedative
(One of the types of drugs used as tranquilizers or sedatives or
hypnotics or muscle relaxants; chronic use can lead to dependency)

Approved for: Treatment of anxiety, to control agitation caused by
alcohol withdrawal, also used to treat irritable bowel syndrome

Dependency and Addiction: Chlordiazepoxide can be habit-
forming. Do not take a larger dose, take it more often, or for a longer
time than your doctor tells you to. Tolerance may develop with
long-term or excessive use, making the drug less effective.

Withdrawals: Stopping the drug suddenly can worsen your
condition and cause withdrawal symptoms such as:

Abdominal cramps
Anxiousness
Convulsions
Dysphoria (a state of anxiety, depression, unease)
Insomnia
Irritability
Muscle cramps
Sleeplessness
Sweating
Tremor
Vomiting

Important Warnings:

In addition to the side effects, precautions and warnings shown on
the label the following have been reported:

Ataxia (Loss of the ability to coordinate muscular movement)
Confusion
Drowsiness

Generic Name: Chlorpromazine
Brand Name: Thorazine

Type or Class of Drug: Chlorpromazine is in a class of medications called conventional antipsychotics

Approved for: Chlorpromazine is used to treat the symptoms of schizophrenia (a mental illness that causes disturbed or unusual thinking, loss of interest in life, and strong or inappropriate emotions) and other psychotic disorders (conditions that cause difficulty telling the difference between things or ideas that are real and things or ideas that are not real) and to treat the symptoms of mania (frenzied, abnormally excited mood) in people who have bipolar disorder (manic depressive disorder; a condition that causes episodes of mania, episodes of depression, and other abnormal moods).

Chlorpromazine is also used to treat severe behavior problems such as explosive, aggressive behavior and hyperactivity in children 1-12 years of age. Chlorpromazine is also used to control nausea and vomiting, to relieve hiccups that have lasted one month or longer, and to relieve restlessness and nervousness that may occur just before surgery.

Chlorpromazine is also used to treat acute intermittent porphyria (condition in which certain natural substances build up in the body and cause stomach pain, changes in thinking and behavior, and other symptoms).

Chlorpromazine is also used along with other medications to treat tetanus (a serious infection that may cause tightening of the muscles, especially the jaw muscle).

Dependency and Addiction: Do not stop taking chlorpromazine without talking to your doctor. Your doctor will probably decrease your dose gradually.

Withdrawals: If you suddenly stop taking chlorpromazine, you may experience withdrawal symptoms, such as:

Dizziness
Gastritis
Nausea
Shakiness
Stomach pain
Tremulousness
Vomiting

Important Warnings:

Both the risk of developing tardive dyskinesia and the likelihood that it will become irreversible are believed to increase as the duration of treatment and the total cumulative dose of antipsychotic drugs administered to the patient increase. However, the syndrome can develop, although much less commonly, after relatively brief treatment periods at low doses.

Studies have shown that older adults with dementia (a brain disorder that affects the ability to remember, think clearly, communicate, and perform daily activities and that may cause changes in mood and personality) who take antipsychotics (medications for mental illness) such as chlorpromazine have an increased chance of death during treatment.

You should know that chlorpromazine may cause dizziness, lightheadedness, fast heartbeat, and fainting, especially when you get up too quickly from a lying position.

Generic Name: Citalopram
Brand Name: Celexa

Type or Class of Drug: Antidepressant

Approved for: Treatment of depression. Sometimes used to treat alcoholism, panic and eating problems.

Dependency and Addiction: Do not stop taking Celexa suddenly. If you do you may experience withdrawal symptoms.

If intolerable symptoms occur following a decrease in dose or upon stopping altogether then a doctor will likely have the patient go back to taking the previous dose and then try reducing the dosage again, this time more gradually.

Withdrawals:
Agitation (suddenly violent and forceful, emotionally disturbed state of mind)
Anxiety
Confusion
Difficulty falling asleep
Difficulty staying asleep
Disturbance of the senses such as electric shock sensations
Dizziness
Dysphoria (a state of anxiety, depression ,unease)
Emotional lability (excessive emotional reactions and frequent mood changes.)
Headache
Hypomania (a state of mind and mood where a person may have excessive energy, little need for sleep, unusual exhilaration, irritability, excitement or aggression)
Insomnia
Irritability
Lethargy
Mood changes
Numbness or tingling in the hands or feet
Parethesias (Paresthesia is a skin sensation such as burning, prickling, itching or tingling with no physical cause. It could be temporary or permanent.)
Tiredness

Important Warnings:

The Black Box Label placed by the FDA on antidepressants including Celexa includes an extensive list of serious, life-threatening potential consequences. There is a tendency among medical professionals and of course with the pharmaceutical and psychiatric industry to downplay these warnings. Don't be fooled. These are real. They do happen and have happened to real people. The FDA does not place warnings like these lightly.

This Black Box Label includes the following warnings. Note that this is not the complete Black Box Label. That can be found at the FDA MedlinePlus website listed in the resources section at the end of this booklet.

* Children, teenagers, and young adults who take antidepressants to treat depression or other mental illnesses may be more likely to become suicidal than children, teenagers, and young adults who do not take antidepressants to treat these conditions.

* You should know that your mental health may change in unexpected ways when you take citalopram or other antidepressants even if you are an adult over 24 years of age. You may become suicidal, especially at the beginning of your treatment and any time that your dose is increased or decreased.

* You, your family, or your caregiver should call your doctor right away if you experience any of the following symptoms: Make sure someone around you such as a family member or friend or caregiver knows these symptoms so they can call the doctor if you are unable to seek treatment on your own.

Acting without thinking
Aggressive behavior
Agitation (suddenly violent and forceful, emotionally disturbed state of mind)
Difficulty falling asleep
Difficulty staying asleep
Extreme worry
Frenxied abnormal excitement

Irritability
New or worsening depression
Panic attacks
Planning to kill yourself
Severe restlessness
Thinking about harming yourself
Thinking about killing yourself
Trying to kill yourself

Generic Name: clonazepam
Brand Name: Klonopin

Type or Class of Drug: benzodiazepine
(One of the types of drugs used as tranquilizers or sedatives or
hypnotics or muscle relaxants; chronic use can lead to dependency)

Approved for: To control certain types of seizures, treat panic
attacks

Dependency and Addiction: Clonazepam can be habit-forming. Do
not take a larger dose, take it more often, or take it for a longer
period of time or in a different way than prescribed by your doctor.

Withdrawals: Your doctor will probably decrease your dose
gradually.

If you suddenly stop taking clonazepam, you may experience
withdrawal symptoms such as:
Anxiety
Changes in behavior
Difficulty falling asleep
Difficulty staying asleep
Hallucinating (seeing things or hearing voices that do not exist)
Muscle cramps
New seizures
Stomach cramps
Sweating
Uncontrollable shaking of a part of your body
Worsening seizures

Important Warnings:

May increase mortality

Cases of sudden death have been reported.

You should know that your mental health may change in unexpected ways, and you may become suicidal (thinking about harming or killing yourself or planning or trying to do so) while you are taking clonazepam

You, your family, or your caregiver should call your doctor right away if you experience any of the following symptoms:

Acting on dangerous impulses
Aggressive behavior
Agitation (suddenly violent and forceful, emotionally disturbed state of mind)
Angry behavior
Anxiety
Any other unusual changes in behavior or mood
Depression
Difficulty falling asleep
Difficulty staying asleep
Giving away prized possessions
Irritability
Mania (frenzied, abnormally excited mood)
New Irritability
Panic attacks
Preoccupation with death or dying
Restlessness
Talking or thinking about wanting to end your life
Talking or thinking about wanting to hurt yourself
Violent behavior
Withdrawing from friends or family
Worsening irritability

Be sure that your family or caregiver knows these symptoms so they can call the doctor if you are unable to seek treatment on your own.

Generic Name: desvenlafaxine
Brand Name: Pristiq

Type or Class of Drug: Antidepressant

Approved for: Depression

Dependency and Addiction: Do not stop taking desvenlafaxine without talking to your doctor. Your doctor will probably decrease your dose gradually.

Withdrawals: If you suddenly stop taking desvenlafaxine, you may experience withdrawal symptoms such as:

Anxiety
Diarrhea
Difficulty falling asleep
Difficulty staying asleep
Dizziness
Extreme tiredness
Headache
Irritability
Nausea
Sweating
Unusual dreams

Tell your doctor if you experience any of these symptoms while you are decreasing your dose of desvenlafaxine or soon after you stop taking desvenlafaxine.

Important Warnings:

The Black Box Label placed by the FDA on antidepressants including Pristiq includes an extensive list of serious, life-threatening potential consequences. There is a tendency among medical professionals and of course with the pharmaceutical and psychiatric industry to downplay these warnings. Don't be fooled. These are real. They do happen and have happened to real people.

The FDA does not place warnings like these lightly.

This Black Box Label includes the following warnings. Note that this is not the complete Black Box Label. That can be found at the FDA MedlinePlus website listed in the resources section at the end of this booklet.

* Children, teenagers, and young adults who take antidepressants to treat depression or other mental illnesses may be more likely to become suicidal than children, teenagers, and young adults who do not take antidepressants to treat these conditions.

* You should know that your mental health may change in unexpected ways when you take citalopram or other antidepressants even if you are an adult over 24 years of age. You may become suicidal, especially at the beginning of your treatment and any time that your dose is increased or decreased.

* You, your family, or your caregiver should call your doctor right away if you experience any of the following symptoms: Make sure someone around you such as a family member or friend or caregiver knows these symptoms so they can call the doctor if you are unable to seek treatment on your own.

Acting without thinking
Aggressive behavior
Agitation (suddenly violent and forceful, emotionally disturbed state of mind)
Difficulty falling asleep
Difficulty staying asleep
Extreme worry
Frenxied abnormal excitement
Irritability
New or worsening depression
Panic attacks
Planning to kill yourself
Severe restlessness
Thinking about harming yourself
Thinking about killing yourself
Trying to kill yourself

May make you drowsy and affect your judgment and thinking.

Generic Name: diazepam
Brand Name: Valium

Type or Class of Drug: Benzodiazepine - minor sedative
(One of the types of drugs used as tranquilizers or sedatives or
hypnotics or muscle relaxants; chronic use can lead to dependency)

Approved for: Used to relieve anxiety, muscle spasms, and seizures
and to control agitation caused by alcohol withdrawal.

Diazepam is also used to treat irritable bowel syndrome and panic
attacks

Dependency and Addiction: Diazepam can be habit-forming. Do
not take a larger dose, take it more often, or for a longer time than
your doctor tells you to. Tolerance may develop with long-term or
excessive use, making the drug less effective. This medication must
be taken regularly to be effective. Do not skip doses even if you feel
that you do not need them. Do not take diazepam for more than 4
months or stop taking this medication without talking to your doctor.

Stopping the drug suddenly can worsen your condition.

Withdrawals: Stopping the drug suddenly can cause withdrawals
such as:

Abdominal cramps
Anxiousness
Convulsions
Irritability
Muscle cramps
Sleeplessness
Sweating
Tremor
Vomiting

Important Warnings:

To assure the safe and effective use of benzodiazepines, patients should be informed that, since benzodiazepines may produce psychological and physical dependence.

Paradoxical reactions (reactions that are the opposite of what is intended) such as the following have been reported:

Anxiety
Hallucinations
Insomnia
Muscle tone increased with an exaggeration of tendon reflexes
Rage
Sleep disturbances
Stimulation
Unusual or excessive excitement

Should these occur, use of this drug should be discontinued.

Please take a good look at all the side effects listed here:
nlm.nih.gov/medlineplus/druginfo/meds/a682047.html#brand-name-1

Generic Name: Diohenoxylate and atropine
Brand Name: Lomotil

Type or Class of Drug: Antidiarrhea

Approved for: Lomotril (Diphenoxylate and atropine) is used to control diarrhea.

Dependency and Addiction: Diphenoxylate can be habit-forming. Do not take a larger dose, take it more often, or for a longer period than your doctor tells you to. Stopping the medicine suddenly after taking it for a long time may cause withdrawal.

Withdrawals:

Muscle cramps
Shaking
Stomach cramps
Trembling
Unusual sweating
Upset stomach
Vomiting

Important Warnings:

You should know that this drug may make you drowsy. Do not drive
a car or operate machinery until you know how this drug affects
you.

Generic Name: duloxetine
Brand Name: Cymbalta

Type or Class of Drug: Antidepressant

Approved for: Depression, Anxiety, fibromyalgia, diabetic
neuropathy

Dependency and Addiction: Do not stop taking duloxetine without
talking to your doctor. Your doctor will probably decrease your dose
gradually. If you suddenly stop taking duloxetine, you may
experience withdrawal symptoms

Withdrawals: Withdrawal symptoms include:

Anxiety
Burning, numbness or tingling in hands or feet
Diarrhea
Difficulty falling asleep
Difficulty staying asleep
Dizziness

Headache
Irritability
Sweating
Nausea
Nightmares
Pain
Tiredness
Vomiting

Important Warnings:

The Black Box Label placed by the FDA on antidepressants including Cymbalta includes an extensive list of serious, life-threatening potential consequences. A tendency exists among medical professionals and of course with the pharmaceutical and psychiatric industry to downplay these warnings. Don't be fooled. These are real. They do happen and have happened to real people. The FDA does not place warnings like these lightly.

This Black Box Label includes the following warnings. Note that this is not the complete Black Box Label. That can be found at the FDA MedlinePlus website listed in the resources section at the end of this booklet.

Cymbalta is not approved for use in pediatric patients

A small number of children, teenagers, and young adults (up to 24 years of age) who took antidepressants ('mood elevators') such as duloxetine during clinical studies became suicidal (thinking about harming or killing oneself or planning or trying to do so).

Children, teenagers, and young adults who take antidepressants to treat depression or other mental illnesses may be more likely to become suicidal than children, teenagers, and young adults who do not take antidepressants to treat these conditions.

You should know that your mental health may change in unexpected ways when you take duloxetine or other antidepressants even if you are an adult over 24 years of age.

These changes may occur even if you do not have a mental illness and you are taking duloxetine to treat a different type of condition.

You may become suicidal taking this drug.

You, your family, or caregiver should call your doctor right away if you experience any of the following symptoms:

Acting without thinking
Aggressive behavior
Agitation (suddenly violent and forceful, emotionally disturbed state of mind)
Behavior changes (any other unusual changes in behavior)
Difficulty falling asleep
Difficulty staying asleep
Extreme worry
Frenzied, abnormal excitement
Hostile behavior
Irritability
New or worsening depression
Panic attacks
Planning or trying to kill yourself
Severe restlessness
Thinking about harming yourself
Thinking about killing yourself

Be sure that your family or caregiver checks on you daily so they can call the doctor if you are unable to seek treatment on your own.

Generic Name: escitalopram
Brand Name: Lexapro

Type or Class of Drug: Antidepressant

Approved for: Treatment of depression, treatment of anxiety

Dependency and Addiction: Do not stop taking escitalopram without talking to your doctor. If you suddenly stop taking escitalopram, you may experience withdrawal symptoms.

Withdrawals: Withdrawals include:

Agitation (suddenly violent and forceful, emotionally disturbed state of mind)
Anxiety
Confusion
Difficulty falling asleep
Difficulty staying asleep
Dizziness
Headache
Irritability
Mood changes
Numbness in hands or feet
Tingling in hands or feet
Tiredness

Important Warnings:

The Black Box Label placed by the FDA on antidepressants including Lexapro includes an extensive list of serious, life-threatening potential consequences. There is a tendency among medical professionals and of course with the pharmaceutical and psychiatric industry to downplay these warnings. Don't be fooled. These are real. They do happen and have happened to real people.

The FDA does not place warnings like these lightly.

This Black Box Label includes the following warnings. Note that this is not the complete Black Box Label. That can be found at the FDA MedlinePlus website listed in the resources section at the end of this booklet.

* Children, teenagers, and young adults who take antidepressants to treat depression or other mental illnesses may be more likely to become suicidal than children, teenagers, and young adults who do not take antidepressants to treat these conditions.

* You should know that your mental health may change in unexpected ways when you take citalopram or other antidepressants even if you are an adult over 24 years of age. You may become suicidal, especially at the beginning of your treatment and any time that your dose is increased or decreased.

* You, your family, or your caregiver should call your doctor right away if you experience any of the following symptoms: Make sure someone around you such as a family member or friend or caregiver knows these symptoms so they can call the doctor if you are unable to seek treatment on your own.

Acting without thinking
Aggressive behavior
Agitation (suddenly violent and forceful, emotionally disturbed state of mind)
Difficulty falling asleep
Difficulty staying asleep
Extreme worry
Frenxied abnormal excitement
Irritability
New or worsening depression
Panic attacks
Planning to kill yourself
Severe restlessness
Thinking about harming yourself
Thinking about killing yourself
Trying to kill yourself

Generic Name: eszopiclone
Brand Name: Lunesta

Type or Class of Drug: Hypnotic

Approved for: Insomnia

Dependency and Addiction: Do not stop taking eszopiclone without talking to your doctor. Your doctor will probably decrease your dose gradually

Withdrawals: . If you suddenly stop taking eszopiclone you may experience withdrawal symptoms such as:

Anxiety
Muscle cramps
Seizures (rarely)
Shakiness
Stomach cramps
Sweating
Unusual dreams
Vomiting

Important Warnings:

Your mental health may change in unexpected ways

Tell your doctor right away if you experience any of the following symptoms:
Aggressiveness
Confusion
Feeling as if you are outside of your body
Hallucinations (seeing things or hearing voices that do not exist)
Memory problems
New depression
Other unusual behavior
Other unusual thoughts
Strange or unusually outgoing behavior
Thinking about killing yourself
Worsening depression

Be sure that your family knows these symptoms so that they can call the doctor if you are unable to seek treatment on your own.

A variety of abnormal thinking and behavior changes have been reported to occur in association with the use of sedative/hypnotics.

Do not engage in hazardous occupations requiring complete mental alertness or motor coordination such as operating machinery or driving a motor vehicle after taking Lunesta. You may suffer these same problems the day after taking this drug.

Generic Name: fentanyl
Brand Name: Actiq and Duragesic

Type or Class of Drug: Opiate (narcotic) pain reliever
A narcotic is a substance that dulls pain and induces sleep. Opiate means that is derived from or acts like opium in dulling the senses and inducing sleep.

Approved for: Breakthrough pain from cancer. Breakthrough pain is sudden episodes of pain that occur despite round the clock treatment with pain medication.

Dependency and Addiction: This drug may become habit-forming, however since Actiq is used for the treatment of chronic cancer pain the National Library of Medicine DailyMed web site recommends that fear of tolerance and physical dependence should not deter using high enough doses to adequately relieve the pain. According to this same web site physical dependence is not ordinarily a concern when one is treating a patient with chronic cancer pain.

Withdrawals:

Do not stop taking Actiq without talking to your doctor. The physical dependence associated with this drug results in withdrawal symptoms in patients who abruptly stop taking Actiq.

Early symptoms of withdrawal include:

Agitation (suddenly violent and forceful, emotionally disturbed state of mind)
Anxiety
Increased tearing
Insomnia
Muscle aches
Runny nose
Sweating
Yawning

Late symptoms of withdrawal include:

Abdominal cramping
Diarrhea
Dilated pupils
Goose bumps
Nausea
Vomiting

Important Warnings: The Black Box Warning * for Actiq includes but is not limited to the following:

Actiq contains a medicine in an amount which can be fatal to a child. Death has been reported in children who have accidentally ingested Actiq.

Actiq is intended to be used only in the care of cancer patients and only by oncologists and pain specialists who are knowledgeable of and skilled in the use of opioids to treat cancer pain. (An opioid is a drug with similar properties to opium. Opioids are drugs used for pain management.)

Opioid painkillers now cause more drug overdose deaths than cocaine and heroin combined.

Information on side effects, overdose symptoms and other special warnings can be found by visiting either of the National Library of Medicine web sites listed in the reference section at the end of this booklet.

Generic Name: fluoxetine
Brand Name: Prozac and Sarafem

Type or Class of Drug: Antidepressant

Approved for: Depression, PMS, eating disorders, panic. OCD. Fluoxetine is also sometimes used to treat alcoholism, attention-deficit disorder, borderline personality disorder, sleep disorders, headaches, mental illness, posttraumatic stress disorder, Tourette's syndrome, obesity, sexual problems, and phobias.

Dependency and Addiction: Do not stop taking without talking to your doctor.

Withdrawals: If you suddenly stop taking fluoxetine, you may experience withdrawal symptoms such as:

Agitiation
Confusion
Dizziness
Difficulty falling asleep
Difficulty staying asleep
Dizziness
Headache
Irritability
Mood changes
Numbness
Tingling in the hands or feet
Tiredness

Important Warnings:

The Black Box Label placed by the FDA on antidepressants including Prozac includes an extensive list of serious, life-threatening potential consequences. There is a tendency among medical professionals and of course with the pharmaceutical and psychiatric industry to downplay these warnings. Don't be fooled. These are real. They do happen and have happened to real people.

The FDA does not place warnings like these lightly.

This Black Box Label includes the following warnings. Note that this is not the complete Black Box Label. That can be found at the FDA MedlinePlus website listed in the resources section at the end of this booklet.

* Children, teenagers, and young adults who take antidepressants to treat depression or other mental illnesses may be more likely to become suicidal than children, teenagers, and young adults who do not take antidepressants to treat these conditions.

* You should know that your mental health may change in unexpected ways when you take Prozac or other antidepressants even if you are an adult over 24 years of age. You may become suicidal, especially at the beginning of your treatment and any time that your dose is increased or decreased.

* You, your family, or your caregiver should call your doctor right away if you experience any of the following symptoms: Make sure someone around you such as a family member or friend or caregiver knows these symptoms so they can call the doctor if you are unable to seek treatment on your own.

Acting without thinking
Aggressive behavior
Agitation (suddenly violent and forceful, emotionally disturbed state of mind)
Difficulty falling asleep
Difficulty staying asleep
Extreme worry
Frenxied abnormal excitement
Irritability
New or worsening depression
Panic attacks
Planning to kill yourself
Severe restlessness
Thinking about harming yourself
Thinking about killing yourself
Trying to kill yourself

May make you drowsy and affect your judgment and thinking.

Generic Name: flurazepam
Brand Name: Dalmane

Type or Class of Drug: Benzodiazepine - Minor Sedative
(One of the types of drugs used as tranquilizers or sedatives or
hypnotics or muscle relaxants; chronic use can lead to dependency)

Approved for: Treatment of Insomnia

Dependency and Addiction: Flurazepam can be habit-forming. Do
not take a larger dose, take it more often, or take it for a longer time
than prescribed by your doctor.
May produce psychological and physical dependence, it is advisable
that they consult with their physician before either increasing the
dose or abruptly discontinuing this drug.

Withdrawals: If you suddenly stop taking flurazepam, especially
after taking it regularly, you may develop withdrawal symptoms
such as:

Difficulty sleeping
Muscle cramps
Sadness
Seizures
Stomach cramps
Sweating
Uncontrollable shaking of part of your body
Vomiting

Important Warnings:

This has not been tested and is not recommended for use in children.

Complex behaviors such as "sleep-driving" (i.e., driving while not
fully awake after ingestion of a sedative-hypnotic, with amnesia for
the event) have been reported.

Other complex behaviors (e.g., preparing and eating food, making phone calls, or having sex) have been reported in patients who are not fully awake after taking a sedative-hypnotic. As with sleep-driving, patients usually do not remember these events.

Patients should also be cautioned about engaging in hazardous occupations requiring complete mental alertness such as operating machinery or driving a motor vehicle after ingesting the drug, including potential impairment of the performance of such activities which may occur the day following ingestion of Flurazepam Hydrochloride Capsules.

Warning for the elderly and debilitated: Dizziness, drowsiness, light-headedness, staggering, ataxia and falling have occurred, particularly in elderly or debilitated persons

Severe sedation, lethargy, disorientation and coma, probably indicative of drug intolerance or overdosage, have been reported.

Other Adverse Reactions that have been reported are:
Anorexia (loss of appetite especially as result of disease)
Apprehension (Fearful or uneasy anticipation of the future; dread.)
Bitter almonds
Blurred vision
Body and joint pains
Burning vision
Chest pains
Confusion
Constipation
Depression
Diarrhea
Difficulty focusing
Dry mouth
Euphoria
Excessive salivation
Faintness
Flushing
Gastrointestinal pain
Genitourinary complaints (of or relating to the genital and urinary organs or their functions.)
Headache

Heartburn
Hallucinations
Hypotension (low blood pressure)
Irritability
Nausea
Nervousness
Palpitations
Pruritus (severe itching, often of normal skin)
Restlessness
Shortness of breath
Skin rash
Slurred speech
Sweating
Talkativeness
Upset stomach
Vomiting
Weakness

Generic Name: haloperidol
Brand Name: Haldol

Type or Class of Drug: antipsychotic

Approved for: Used to treat psychotic disorders, Tourette's disorder, severe behavioral problems such as explosive, aggressive behavior or hyperactivity in children who cannot be treated with psychotherapy or with other medications

Dependancy and Addiction: Your doctor will probably decrease your dose gradually. If you suddenly stop taking haloperidol, you may experience difficulty controlling your movements.

Withdrawals: If you suddenly stop taking haloperidol, you may experience difficulty controlling your movements.

Important Warnings:

Tardive dyskinesia, a syndrome consisting of potentially irreversible, involuntary, dyskinetic movements, may appear in some patients on long-term therapy or may occur after drug therapy has been discontinued. The syndrome is characterized by rhythmical involuntary movements of tongue, face, mouth or jaw (e.g., protrusion of tongue, puffing of cheeks, puckering of mouth, chewing movements). Sometimes these may be accompanied by involuntary movements of extremities and the trunk.

The following have been reported in connection with taking Haldol:

Agitation (suddenly violent and forceful, emotionally disturbed state of mind)
Anxiety
Catatonic-like behavioral (state in which a person does not move or speak at all or moves or speaks abnormally)
Confusion
Depression
Drowsiness
Euphoria
Gand mal seizures
Hallucinations
Headache
Insomnia
Lethargy
Restlessness
Worsening of psychotic symptoms

May cause heart failure or sudden death.

Treatment with antipsychotic drugs may increase mortality.

Generic Name: hydrocodone and acetaminophen
Brand Name: Lorcet

Type or Class of Drug: Opiate (narcotic) pain killer
A narcotic is a substance that dulls pain and induces sleep. Opiate
means that is derived from or acts like opium in dulling the senses
and inducing sleep.

Approved for: Treatment of pain and coughing

Dependency and Addiction: Hydrocodone may be habit-forming.
Take hydrocodone exactly as directed. Do not take a larger dose,
take it more often, or take it for a longer period of time than
prescribed by your doctor. Call your doctor if you develop a strong
desire to take more medication than prescribed.

The acetaminophen part of this drug is not habit forming however it
does have side effects and serious overdose cautions. Please see
FDA MedlinePlus web site referenced at the end of this booklet for
more information.

Withdrawals: If you suddenly stop taking hydrocodone, you may
experience withdrawal symptoms.

Anxiety
Back pain
Chills
Cravings
Depression
Diarrhea
Fatigue
Feeling sick
Flu-like symptoms
Insomnia
Irritability
Loss of apetite
Muscle aches
Muscle pains
Runny nose

Sleep disturbances
Sweating
Watery eyes
Yawning

Important Warnings:

"Doctor shopping" to obtain additional prescriptions is common among drug abusers and people suffering from untreated addiction.

Call your doctor if your symptoms are not controlled by the hydrocodone product you are taking. Do not increase your dose of medication on your own.

Hydrocodone may make you drowsy. Do not drive a car or operate machinery until you know how this medication affects you.

Generic Name: Hydromorphone
Brand Name: Dilaudid

Type or Class of Drug: Pain reliever

Approved for: Relieve moderate to severe pain. May also be used to decrease coughing.

Dependancy and Addiction: Hydromorphone can be habit-forming. Do not take a larger dose, take it more often, or for a longer period than your doctor tells you to.

Withdrawals: Physical dependence results in withdrawal symptoms in patients who abruptly discontinue the drug. Withdrawal symptoms include:

Abdominal cramps
Acute withdrawal syndrome
Anorexia (loss of appetite especially as result of disease)
Anxiety
Backache
Chills

Diarrhea
Increased blood pressure
Increased heart rate
Increased respiratory rate
Insomnia
Irritability
Joint pain
Lacrimation (watery eyes)
Myalgia (muscular pain or tenderness)
Mydriasis (prolonged and abnormal dilation (expanding, getting
larger) of the pupil often due to drugs)
Perspiration
Restlessness
Runny nose
Vomiting
Weakness
Yawning

Important Warnings:

Infants born to mothers physically dependent on DILAUDID will
also be physically dependent and may exhibit respiratory difficulties
and withdrawal symptoms.

Adverse reactions to this drug include:

The major hazards of Dilauded are respiratory depression and apnea
(breathing that slows or stops from any cause).

Other hazards include:

Cardiac arrest
Circulatory depression
Dizziness
Dry mouth
Dysphoria (a state of anxiety, depression ,unease)
Euphoria
Flushing
Light-headedness
Nausea
Pruritus

Respiratory arrest
Sedation
Shock
Sweating
Vomiting

Risk of respiratory depression that might result in death

Generic Name: lisdexamfetamine
Brand Name: Vyvance

Type or Class of Drug: Central Nervous System Stimulant
[A stimulant is a drug that increases heart rate, breathing rate, brain function. And nervous system.]

Approved for: ADHD

Dependency and Addiction: Lisdexamfetamine can be habit-forming. Do not take a larger dose, take it more often, take it for a longer time, or take it in a different way than prescribed by your doctor. If you take too much lisdexamfetamine, you may find that the medication no longer controls your symptoms, you may feel a need to take large amounts of the medication, and you may experience symptoms such as rash, difficulty falling asleep or staying asleep, irritability, hyperactivity, and unusual changes in your personality or behavior. Overusing lisdexamfetamine may also cause sudden death or serious heart problems, such as heart attack or stroke.

Withdrawals:

Your doctor will probably decrease your dose gradually and monitor you carefully during this time.

If you suddenly stop taking Vyvanse you may develop:
Extreme tiredness
Severe depression

Important Warnings:

Overusing lisdexamfetamine may also cause sudden death or serious heart problems, such as heart attack or stroke.

Chronic use and dependence may result in:

Hyperactivity (a condition characterized by excessive restlessness and movement)
Insomnia
Irritability
Personality changes
Psychosis
Schizophrenia
Skin disease

You should know that this medication may make it difficult for you to perform activities that require alertness or physical coordination. Do not drive a car or operate machinery until you know how this medication affects you.

Generic Name: lorazepam
Brand Name: Ativan

Type or Class of Drug: Benzodiazepine - Minor Sedative
(One of the types of drugs used as tranquilizers or sedatives or hypnotics or muscle relaxants; chronic use can lead to dependency)

Approved for: Relieving anxiety. It's also used to treat irritable bowel syndrome, epilepsy, insomnia, and nausea and vomiting from cancer treatment and to control agitation caused by alcohol withdrawal.

Dependency and Addiction: Lorazepam can be habit-forming. Do not take a larger dose, take it more often, or for a longer time than your doctor tells you to. Tolerance may develop with long-term or excessive use, making the drug less effective. Do not take lorazepam for more than 4 months or stop taking this medication without talking to your doctor.

Withdrawals:

Do not suddenly stop taking this drug. Stopping the drug suddenly can worsen your condition. You will need to come off this drug gradually in order to control the withdrawal symptoms which include:

Abdominal cramps
Agitation (suddenly violent and forceful, emotionally disturbed state of mind)
Anxiety
Anxiousness
Confusion
Convulsions
Delirium (a temporary state of extreme mental confusion which can include anxiety, disorientation, hallucinations, delusions, and incoherent speech.
Depression
Depersonalization (feeling of no longer being an individual or no longer being yourself - feeling of watching oneself act and having no control over what one is doing)
Derealization (condition where the external world seems strange or unreal)
Diarrhea
Dizziness
Dysphoria (a state of anxiety, depression ,unease)
Hallucinations
Headache
Hyperacusis (Impaired ability to tolerate normal environmental sounds)
Hyperreflexia (overactive or over-responsive reflexes. Examples can include twitching or spastic tendencies)
Hypersensitivity to light (hyper means exaggerated or too much, extreme, above normal)
Hypersensitivity to noise (hyper means exaggerated or too much, extreme, above normal)
Hypersensitivity to perceptual changes (hyper means exaggerated or too much, extreme, above normal)

Hypersensitivity to physical contact (hyper means exaggerated or too much, extreme, above normal)
Hyperthermia (abnormally high body temperature usually the result of head injury, medication or infection)
Insomnia
Involuntary movements
Irritability
Loss of appetite
Myalgia (muscle pain)
Nausea
Numbness of extremities
Palpitations (heartbeat sensations that feel like your heart is pounding or racing)
Panic attacks
Rebound phenomena (the tendency of a medication, when discontinued, to cause a return of the symptoms being treated to be more severe than before)
Restlessness
Seizures
Short term memory loss
Sleeplessness
Sweating
Tachycardia (a rapid heart rate)
Tension
Tingling of extremities
Tremors
Vertigo
Vomiting

Some symptoms of Ativan withdrawal have not been listed on the government web sites used as primary research for this booklet. More symptoms of Ativan withdrawal can be found at: http://www.prozactruth.com/ativan.htm

Do not suddenly stop taking Ativan. Your doctor probably will decrease your dose gradually.

Important Warnings:

In patients who are depressed a possibility for suicide should be borne in mind.

Lorazepam should be used with caution in patients with any sort of respiratory (breathing) or lung problems.

Special caution, elderly or debilitated patients may be more susceptible to the sedative effects of Ativan (lorazepam). Sedative means the reduction of anxiety, stress, irritability, or excitement.

Paradoxical reactions have occasionally been reported during use. (A paradoxical reaction is one which is the opposite of what is expected or intended.) These reactions are more likely to occur in children and the elderly. Should this occur, use of the drug should be stopped. A paradoxical reaction is when the drug produces the opposite effect as is expected. So if a person has a paradoxical reaction to a drug that is supposed to have a calming affect the drug will instead produce anxiety.

Generic Name: meperidine
Brand Name: Demerol and Mepergan

Type or Class of Drug: Narcotic pain reliever (a group of pain medications similar to morphine)

Approved for: Relieve moderate to severe pain

Dependency and Addiction: Meperidine can be habit-forming. Do not take a larger dose, or take it more often or for a longer period of time than you were told by your doctor. Your doctor will want to reduce your dosage gradually.

Withdrawals: Withdrawal symptoms may include:

Abdominal cramps
Anorexia (loss of appetite especially as result of disease)
Anxiety
Back pain
Chills
Diarrhea
Fast breathing
Fast heart rate
Increased blood pressure
Increased heart rate
Increased respiratory rate
Insomnia
Irritability
Joint pain
Loss of appetite
Muscle pain
Myalgia (muscular pain or tenderness)
Mydriasis (prolonged and abnormal dilation (expanding, getting larger) of the pupil often due to drugs)
Nausea
Nervousness
Restlessness
Stomach pain
Stuffy nose
Sweating
Upset stomach
Vomiting
Watery eyes
Weakness
Yawning

Important Warnings:

Alcohol and street drugs can make the side effects from meperidine worse and can cause serious harm or death.

Do not drive a car or operate machinery until you know how this medication affects you.

The major hazards of meperidine are:

Cardiac arrest
Circulatory depression
Respiratory arrest
Respiratory depression (trouble breathing)
Shock

The most frequently observed adverse reactions include:
Dizziness
Lightheadedness
Nausea
Sedation
Sweating
Vomiting

Generic Name: methylphenidate
Brand Name: Ritalin

Type or Class of Drug: Central Nervous System Stimulant
[A stimulant is a drug that increases heart rate, breathing rate, brain function. And nervous system.]

Approved for: ADHD and Narcolepsy

Dependency and Addiction: Methylphenidate can be habit-forming. Methylphenidate can be habit-forming. Do not take a larger dose, take it more often, take it for a longer time, or take it in a different way than prescribed by your doctor. If you take too much methylphenidate, you may find that the medication no longer controls your symptoms, you may feel a need to take large amounts of the medication, and you may experience unusual changes in your behavior

Withdrawals:

Do not stop taking methylphenidate without talking to your doctor. The main withdrawal symptoms noted are:

Severe depression
Extreme fatigue
Changes in heart rhythm.

Important Warnings:

Methylphenidate may cause sudden death in children and teenagers, especially children or teenagers with heart defects or serious heart problems.

This medication also may cause sudden death, heart attack or stroke in adults, especially adults with heart defects or serious heart problems.

Methylphenidate may slow children's growth or weight gain.

Stimulants such as methylphenidate create a rise in blood pressure.

Stimulants may make any problems with behavior or problems a person is having with their thoughts worse than they were before taking the medication.

Aggressive behavior or hostility has been seen in connection with the taking of stimulants. This behavior should be watched for in patients taking methylphenidate.

Psychotic and manic symptoms such as hallucinations or delusional thinking can be caused by this drug in patients who have had not previous history of these feelings and problems. This can occur at just normal doses prescribed by a doctor.

Difficulty focusing and blurring of vision have been reported in people taking stimulant drugs such as Concerta.

There is some evidence stimulants may cause seizures.

Other adverse reactions to stimulants include:

Anxiety
Blood pressure increased
Decreased appetite
Dizziness
Dry mouth
Headache
Hyperhidrosis (excessive sweating)
Insomnia
Irritability
Nausea
Upper abdominal pain
Weight decreased

Generic Name: Modafinil
Brand Name: Provigil

Type or Class of Drug: Wakefulness promoting agent

Approved for: Treatment of narcolepsy (a condition that causes excessive daytime sleepiness). Sometimes used for other sleep problems.

Dependency and Addiction: Modafinil may be habit-forming. Do not take a larger dose, take it more often, or take it for a longer period of time than prescribed by your doctor.

This drug can lead to dependence and has been known to be abused.

Withdrawals:

No specific withdrawals were observed during a trial however sleepiness returned in narcoleptic patients.

Feeling the need to continue taking the drug (addiction).

Important Warnings:

Modafinil should not be used in place of getting enough sleep
You should know that modafinil may affect your judgment or thinking.
Provigil (modafinil) may not completely relieve the sleepiness caused by your disorder
Do not drive a car or operate machinery until you know how this medication affects you.
Provigil cannot cure sleep disorders and it may not stop all of your sleepiness.

Generic Name: morphine
Brand Name: Roxanol and Duramorph

Type or Class of Drug: Opiate (narcotic) pain reliever
A narcotic is a substance that dulls pain and induces sleep. Opiate means that is derived from or acts like opium in dulling the senses and inducing sleep.

Approved for: Treating moderate to severe pain

Dependency and Addiction: Morphine can be habit-forming. Take morphine exactly as directed. Do not take a larger dose, take it more often, or take it for a longer period of time or in a different way than prescribed by your doctor.
Physical dependence and tolerance are not unusual.

Withdrawals: Should not be abruptly discontinued. Do not stop taking morphine without talking to your doctor. Your doctor may decrease your dose gradually. If you suddenly stop taking morphine, you may experience withdrawal symptoms such as:

Abdominal cramps
Anorexia (loss of appetite especially as result of disease)
Anxiety
Backache
Chills
Coughing

Diarrhea
Difficulty falling asleep
Difficulty staying asleep
Hair on your skin standing on end
Hallucinating (seeing things or hearing voices that do not exist)
Increased blood pressure
Increased heart rate
Increased respiratory rate
Insomnia
Irritability
Joint pain
Myalgia (muscular pain or tenderness)
Mydriasis (prolonged and abnormal dilation (expanding, getting larger) of the pupil often due to drugs)
Nausea
Perspiration
Restlessness
Runny nose
Shaking of a part of your body that you cannot control
Sneezing
Sweating
Vomiting
Watery eyes
Weakness
Yawning

Important Warnings:

Morphine may cause dizziness, lightheadedness, and fainting when you get up too quickly from a lying position.

Ingestion of these capsules or of the pellets within the capsules may cause fatal respiratory depression when administered to patients not already tolerant to high doses of opioids.

Generic Name: olanzapine
Brand Name: Zyprexa

Type or Class of Drug: Antipsychotic

Approved for: To treat the symptoms of schizophrenia. It is also used to treat bipolar disorder

Dependency and Addiction: Do not stop taking olanzapine without talking to your doctor. Your doctor will probably want to decrease your dose gradually.

Withdrawals:

Zyprexa withdrawal symptoms can include, but are not limited to:

Being suspicious
Being withdrawn
Believing things that aren't true
Delusions
Depression
Hallucinations (seeing or hearing things that aren't there)
Hearing voices
Insomnia
Mania
Symptoms of schizophrenia

Important Warnings:

The risk of developing tardive dyskinesia and the likelihood that it will become irreversible are believed to increase as the duration of treatment and the total cumulative dose of antipsychotic drugs administered to the patient increase. However, the syndrome can develop, although much less commonly, after relatively brief treatment periods at low doses or may even arise after discontinuation of treatment.

Older adults with dementia may also have a greater chance of having a stroke or mini-stroke during treatment. If you experience any of the following symptoms, call your doctor immediately: slow or difficult speech, sudden dizziness or faintness, or weakness or numbness of an arm or leg.

You should know that olanzapine may cause fast or slow heartbeat, dizziness, lightheadedness, and fainting when you get up too quickly from a lying position.

Teenagers who take olanzapine are more likely than adults who take olanzapine to gain weight, have increased levels of fat in their blood, develop liver problems, and experience side effects such as sleepiness, breast enlargement, and discharge from the breasts.

Generic Name: oxycodone
Brand Name: Oxycontin, part of Percocet and Percodan

Type or Class of Drug: Opiate (narcotic) pain killer
A narcotic is a substance that dulls pain and induces sleep. Opiate means that is derived from or acts like opium in dulling the senses and inducing sleep.

Approved for: Relief of moderate to severe pain

Dependency and Addiction: Oxycodone can be habit-forming. Do not take a larger dose, take it more often, or take it for a longer period of time than prescribed by your doctor. If you have been taking oxycodone for more than a few days, do not stop taking oxycodone suddenly.

Oxycodone can produce drug dependence of the morphine type and, therefore, has the potential for being abused.

Withdrawals: If you stop taking this medication suddenly, you may experience withdrawal symptoms such as:

Anxiety
Chills
Cramps
Depression
Diarrhea
Difficulty falling asleep
Difficulty staying asleep
Fast breathing
Fast heartbeat
Irritability
Joint aches or pains
Loss of appetite
Muscle aches or pains
Nausea
Restlessness
Runny nose
Sneezing
Sweating
Vomiting
Watery eyes
Weakness
Yawning

Call your doctor if you have any withdrawal symptoms when your dose is decreased or when you stop taking oxycodone.

Important Warnings:
You should know that this medication may make you drowsy. Do not drive a car, operate heavy machinery, or participate in any other possibly dangerous activities until you know how this medication affects you.

Oxycodone may cause dizziness, lightheadedness, and fainting when you get up too quickly from a lying position.

See label or MedlinePlus web site for the full list of side effects and other warnings.

Generic Name: paroxetine
Brand Name: Paxil

Type or Class of Drug: Antidepressant

Approved for: Used to treat depression, panic disorder (sudden, unexpected attacks of extreme fear and worry about these attacks), and social anxiety disorder (extreme fear of interacting with others or performing in front of others that interferes with normal life).

Paroxetine is also sometimes used to treat chronic headaches, tingling in the hands and feet caused by diabetes, and certain male sexual problems

Are also used to treat obsessive-compulsive disorder (bothersome thoughts that won't go away and the need to perform certain actions over and over), generalized anxiety disorder (GAD; excessive worrying that is difficult to control), and posttraumatic stress disorder (disturbing psychological symptoms that develop after a frightening experience). Paroxetine extended-release tablets are also used to treat premenstrual dysphoric disorder (PMDD, physical and psychological symptoms that occur before the onset of the menstrual period each month).

Dependency and Addiction: Do not stop taking paroxetine without talking to your doctor. Your doctor will probably decrease your dose gradually.

Withdrawals: If you suddenly stop taking paroxetine, you may experience withdrawal symptoms such as:

Abnormally excited mood
Anxiety
Confusion
Depression
Difficulty falling asleep
Difficulty staying asleep
Dizziness
Frenzied mood
Headache
Irritability

Mood changes
Nausea
Numbness in arms, legs, hands or feet
Sweating
Tingling in arms, legs, hands or feet
Tiredness
Unusual dreams

Tell your doctor if you experience any of these symptoms when your dose of paroxetine is decreased.

Important Warnings:

The Black Box Label placed by the FDA on antidepressants including Paxil includes an extensive list of serious, life-threatening potential consequences. There is a tendency among medical professionals and of course with the pharmaceutical and psychiatric industry to downplay these warnings. Don't be fooled. These are real. They do happen and have happened to real people. The FDA does not place warnings like these lightly.

This Black Box Label includes the following warnings. Note that this is not the complete Black Box Label. That can be found at the FDA MedlinePlus website listed in the resources section at the end of this booklet.

* Children, teenagers, and young adults who take antidepressants to treat depression or other mental illnesses may be more likely to become suicidal than children, teenagers, and young adults who do not take antidepressants to treat these conditions.

* You should know that your mental health may change in unexpected ways when you take citalopram or other antidepressants even if you are an adult over 24 years of age. You may become suicidal, especially at the beginning of your treatment and any time that your dose is increased or decreased.

* You, your family, or your caregiver should call your doctor right away if you experience any of the following symptoms: Make sure someone around you such as a family member or friend or caregiver knows these symptoms so they can call the doctor if you are unable to seek treatment on your own.

Acting without thinking
Aggressive behavior
Agitation (suddenly violent and forceful, emotionally disturbed state of mind)
Difficulty falling asleep
Difficulty staying asleep
Extreme worry
Frenxied abnormal excitement
Irritability
New or worsening depression
Panic attacks
Planning to kill yourself
Severe restlessness
Thinking about harming yourself
Thinking about killing yourself
Trying to kill yourself

May make you drowsy and affect your judgment and thinking.

Generic Name: Pregabalin
Brand Name: Lyrica

Type or Class of Drug: Anticonvulsant

Approved for: To treat pain from damaged nerves if you have Diabetes. It is also used to treat pain from shingles and is used to treat certain types of epileptic seizures. Used to treat pain associated with fibromyalgia.

Dependency and Addiction: Pregabalin may be habit forming. Do not take a larger dose, take it more often, or take it for a longer period of time than prescribed by your doctor.

Withdrawals: If you suddenly stop taking pregabalin, you may experience withdrawal symptoms including:

Diarrhea
Headaches
Nausea
Seizures
Trouble falling alseep
Trouble staying asleep

Important Warnings:

Your mental health may change in unexpected ways and you may become suicidal from taking this medication.

You or your family or care giver should notify your doctor right away if you experience any of the following:

Acting on dangerous impulses
Aggressiveness
Agitation (suddenly violent and forceful, emotionally disturbed state of mind)
Anger
Anxiety
Depression
Difficulty falling asleep
Difficulty staying asleep
Giving away prized posessions
Mania (frenzied, abnormally excited mood);
New irritability
Panic attacks
Preoccupation with death and dying
Restlessness
Talking about wanting to hurt yourself or end your life
Thinking about wanting to hurt yourself or end your life
Thinking of killing yourself or planning to do so
Trying to kill yourself
Unusual changes in behavior or mood
Violent behavior
Withdrawing from friends and family
Worsening irritability

Be sure that your family or caregiver knows these symptoms so they can call the doctor if you are unable to seek treatment on your own.

Generic: propoxyphene
Brand: Darvon

Type or Class of Drug: Pain Reliever - opioid

Approved for: Treat mild to moderate pain

Dependency and Addiction: This drug can be habit-forming. Do not take a larger dose, take it more often, or for a longer period than your doctor tells you to. Should not be abruptly discontinued.

Withdrawals: Withdrawal symptoms for Darvon include some or all of the following:

Abdominal cramps
Anorexia (loss of appetite especially as result of disease)
Anxiety
Backache
Chills
Diarrhea
Increased blood pressure
Increased heart rate
Increased respiratory rate
Insomnia
Irritability
Joint pain
Lacrimation (watery eyes)
Myalgia (muscular pain or tenderness)
Mydriasis (prolonged and abnormal dilation (expanding, getting larger) of the pupil often due to drugs)
Nausea
Restlessness
Runny nose
Sweating
Vomiting
Weakness
Yawning

Important Warnings:

There have been numerous cases of accidental and intentional overdose connected with Darvocet alone or in combination with other drugs.

Do not take Darvon (propoxyphene) in combination with other drugs that cause drowsiness: alcohol, tranquilizers, sleep aids, antidepressant drugs, or antihistamines.

Fatalities within the first hour of over-dosage are not uncommon.

Patients should be advised that Darvon may impair mental and/or physical ability required for the performance of potentially hazardous tasks (e.g., driving, operating heavy machinery).

Should not be prescribed for patients who are suicidal or have a history of suicidal ideation.

May cause high blood pressure.

May cause respiratory depression especially in the elderly and the debilitated. (respiratory depression is breathing that is slower than normal or which fails to fill the lungs as well as normal)

During the clinical trials where this drug was tested the reported adverse reactions included:

Abdominal pain
Constipation
Dizziness
Dysphoria (a state of anxiety, depression ,unease)
Euphoria
Hallucinations
Headache
Lightheadedness
Minor visual disturbances
Nausea
Sedation
Skin rashes
Vomiting

Weakness

Since Darvon has been on the market the most frequently reported adverse events have included:

Accidental overdose
Cardiac arrest
Cardio-respiratory arrest
Coma
Completed suicide
Confusional state
Convulsions
Death
Diarrhea
Dizziness
Drug dependence
Drug ineffective
Drug toxicity
Intentional overdose
Nausea
Respiratory arrest
Vomiting

Opioid painkillers now cause more drug overdose deaths than cocaine and heroin combined.

Generic Name: quetiapine
Brand Name: Seroquel

Type or Class of Drug: Antipsychotic

Approved for: Treatment of schizophrenia (a mental illness that causes disturbed or unusual thinking, loss of interest in life, and strong or inappropriate emotions).
Also used to treat mania, depression, bipolar disorder and to treat schizophrenia and bipolar disorder in children. (However see the FDA's Black Label Warning before allowing this to be given to your child)

Dependency and Addiction: Do not stop taking quetiapine without talking to your doctor. Your doctor will probably want to decrease your dose gradually.

Withdrawals: If you suddenly stop taking quetiapine, you may experience withdrawal symptoms such as:

Diarrhea
Difficulty falling asleep
Difficulty staying asleep
Dizziness
Headache
Insomnia
Irritability
Nausea
Vomiting

Important Warnings: The Black Box Label placed by the FDA on antidepressants including quetiapine includes an extensive list of serious, life-threatening potential consequences. There is a tendency among medical professionals and of course with the pharmaceutical and psychiatric industry to downplay these warnings. Don't be fooled. These are real. They do happen and have happened to real people. The FDA does not place warnings like these lightly.

This Black Box Label includes the following warnings. Note that this is not the complete Black Box Label. That can be found at the FDA MedlinePlus website listed in the resources section at the end of this booklet.

* Children, teenagers, and young adults who take antidepressants to treat depression or other mental illnesses may be more likely to become suicidal than children, teenagers, and young adults who do not take antidepressants to treat these conditions.

* You should know that your mental health may change in unexpected ways when you take quetiapine or other antidepressants even if you are an adult over 24 years of age. You may become suicidal, especially at the beginning of your treatment and any time that your dose is increased or decreased.

* You, your family, or your caregiver should call your doctor right away if you experience any of the following symptoms: Make sure someone around you such as a family member or friend or caregiver knows these symptoms so they can call the doctor if you are unable to seek treatment on your own.

Acting without thinking
Aggressive behavior
Agitation (suddenly violent and forceful, emotionally disturbed state of mind)
Difficulty falling asleep
Difficulty staying asleep
Extreme worry
Frenxied abnormal excitement
Irritability
New or worsening depression
Panic attacks
Planning to kill yourself
Severe restlessness
Thinking about harming yourself
Thinking about killing yourself
Trying to kill yourself

The risk of developing tardive dyskinesia and the likelihood that it will become irreversible are believed to increase as the duration of treatment and the total cumulative dose of antipsychotic drugs administered to the patient increase. However, the syndrome can develop, although much less commonly, after relatively brief treatment periods at low doses or may even arise after discontinuation of treatment.

Studies have shown that older adults with dementia (a brain disorder that affects the ability to remember, think clearly, communicate, and perform daily activities and that may cause changes in mood and personality) who take antipsychotics (medications for mental illness) such as quetiapine have an increased risk of death during treatment.

You should know that quetiapine may make it harder for your body to cool down when it gets very hot.

Generic Name: risperidone
Brand Name: Risperdal

Type or Class of Drug: Antipsychotic

Approved for: Schizophrenia (a mental illness that causes disturbed or unusual thinking, loss of interest in life, and strong or inappropriate emotions) in adults and teenagers 13 years of age and older. It is also used to treat episodes of mania (frenzied, abnormally excited, or irritated mood) or mixed episodes (symptoms of mania and depression that happen together) in adults and in teenagers and children 10 years of age and older with bipolar disorder (manic depressive disorder; a disease that causes episodes of depression, episodes of mania, and other abnormal moods).

Risperidone is also used to treat behavior problems such as aggression, self-injury, and sudden mood changes in teenagers and children 5-16 years of age who have autism (a condition that causes repetitive behavior, difficulty interacting with others, and problems with communication).

Dependency and Addiction: Do not stop taking risperidone without talking to your doctor. If you suddenly stop taking risperidone, your symptoms may return and your illness may become harder to treat.

Withdrawals:

Delusions
Depression
Hallucinations
Insomnia
Irritability

Important Warnings:

The risk of developing tardive dyskinesia and the likelihood that it will become irreversible are believed to increase as the duration of treatment and the total cumulative dose of antipsychotic drugs administered to the patient increase. However, the syndrome can develop, although much less commonly, after relatively brief treatment periods at low doses.

Generic Name: secobarbital
Brand Name: Seconal

Type or Class of Drug: Barbiturate

Approved for: Used on a short-term basis to treat insomnia (difficulty falling asleep or staying asleep), also used to treat anxiety before surgery

Dependency and Addiction: Do not stop taking secobarbital without talking to your doctor. Your doctor will probably decrease your dose gradually.

Secobarbital should normally be taken for short periods of time. If you take secobarbital for 2 weeks or longer, secobarbital may not help you sleep as well as it did when you first began to take the medication. If you take secobarbital for a long time, you may also develop dependence ('addiction,' a need to continue taking the medication) on secobarbital.

Talk to your doctor about the risks of taking secobarbital for 2 weeks or longer. Do not take a larger dose of secobarbital, take it more often, or take it for a longer time than prescribed by your doctor.

Withdrawals: If you suddenly stop taking secobarbital, you may develop:

Anxiety
Changes in vision
Difficulty falling asleep
Difficulty staying asleep
Dizziness
Muscle twitching
Nausea
Uncontrollable shaking of your hands or fingers
Vomiting
Weakness

Or you may experience more severe withdrawal symptoms such as seizures or extreme confusion.

Important Warnings:

You should know that some people who took medications for sleep got out of bed and drove their cars, prepared and ate food, had sex, made phone calls, or were involved in other activities while partially asleep. After they woke up, these people were usually unable to remember what they had done.

Call your doctor right away if you find out that you have been driving or doing anything else while you were sleeping.

You should know that this medication may make you drowsy during the daytime. Do not drive a car or operate machinery until you know how this medication affects you.

Generic Name: sertraline
Brand Name: Zoloft

Type or Class of Drug: Antidepressant

Approved for: Sertraline is used to treat depression, obsessive-compulsive disorder (bothersome thoughts that won't go away and the need to perform certain actions over and over), panic attacks (sudden, unexpected attacks of extreme fear and worry about these attacks), posttraumatic stress disorder (disturbing psychological symptoms that develop after a frightening experience), and social anxiety disorder (extreme fear of interacting with others or performing in front of others that interferes with normal life). It is also used to relieve the symptoms of premenstrual dysphoric disorder, including mood swings, irritability, bloating, and breast tenderness. Sertraline is also used sometimes to treat headaches and sexual problems.

Dependency and Addiction: Do not stop taking sertraline without talking to your doctor.

Withdrawals:

Abdominal pain
Agitation (suddenly violent and forceful, emotionally disturbed state of mind)
Anxiety
Diarrhea
Dizziness
Dry Mouth
Dyspepsia
Ejaculation failure
Fatigue
Headache
Hot flush
Insomnia
Nausea
Nervousness
Palpitations
Somnolence
Tremors

Important Warnings:

The Black Box Label placed by the FDA on antidepressants including bupropion includes an extensive list of serious, life-threatening potential consequences. There is a tendency among medical professionals and of course with the pharmaceutical and psychiatric industry to downplay these warnings. Don't be fooled. These are real. They do happen and have happened to real people. The FDA does not place warnings like these lightly.

This Black Box Label includes the following warnings. Note that this is not the complete Black Box Label. That can be found at the FDA MedlinePlus website listed in the resources section at the end of this booklet.

* Children, teenagers, and young adults who take antidepressants to treat depression or other mental illnesses may be more likely to become suicidal than children, teenagers, and young adults who do not take antidepressants to treat these conditions.

* You should know that your mental health may change in unexpected ways when you take bupropion or other antidepressants even if you are an adult over 24 years of age. You may become suicidal, especially at the beginning of your treatment and any time that your dose is increased or decreased.

* You, your family, or your caregiver should call your doctor right away if you experience any of the following symptoms: Make sure someone around you such as a family member or friend or caregiver knows these symptoms so they can call the doctor if you are unable to seek treatment on your own.

Acting without thinking
Aggressive behavior
Agitation (suddenly violent and forceful, emotionally disturbed state of mind)
Difficulty falling asleep
Difficulty staying asleep
Extreme worry
Frenxied abnormal excitement
Irritability
New or worsening depression
Panic attacks
Planning to kill yourself
Severe restlessness
Thinking about harming yourself
Thinking about killing yourself
Trying to kill yourself

Generic Name: temazepam
Brand Name: Restoril

Type or Class of Drug: Benzodiazepine - minor sedative
(One of the types of drugs used as tranquilizers or sedatives or
hypnotics or muscle relaxants; chronic use can lead to dependency)

Approved for: Used on a short-term basis to treat insomnia
(difficulty falling asleep or staying asleep).

Dependency and Addiction: Talk to your doctor before you stop
taking this medication. Your doctor will probably decrease your
dose gradually. Impaired control over drug use, compulsive use,
continued use despite harm, and craving

Withdrawals: If you suddenly stop taking temazepam, you may
experience the following:

Depression
Difficulty falling asleep
Difficulty staying asleep
Muscle cramps
Seizures (rarely)
Stomach cramps
Sweating
Uncontrollable shaking of a part of the body
Vomiting

Important Warnings:

Tell your doctor right away if you experience any of the following
symptoms:

Aggressive
Confusion
Difficulty concentrating
Feeling as if you are outside of your body
Hallucinations (seeing things or hearing voices that do not exist)
Memory problems
New depression

Other changes in your usual thoughts, mood or behavior
Strange or unusually outgoing behavior
Suicidal thoughts
Thinking about killing yourself
Worsening depression

Be sure that your family knows these symptoms so that they can call the doctor if you are unable to seek treatment on your own.

Generic Name: trazodone
Brand Name: Desyrel

Type or Class of Drug: Antidepressant

Approved for: Trazodone is used to treat depression. Sometimes prescribed for insomnia and schizophrenia.

Dependency and Addiction: None mentioned in labeling. However, do not stop taking without checking with your doctor.

Withdrawals: Do not stop taking trazodone without talking to your doctor. Your doctor will probably decrease your dose gradually.

Important Warnings:

The Black Box Label placed by the FDA on antidepressants including Cymbalta includes an extensive list of serious, life-threatening potential consequences. There is a tendency among medical professionals and of course with the pharmaceutical and psychiatric industry to downplay these warnings. Don't be fooled. These are real. They do happen and have happened to real people. The FDA does not place warnings like these lightly.

This Black Box Label includes the following warnings. Note that this is not the complete Black Box Label. That can be found at the FDA MedlinePlus website listed in the resources section at the end of this booklet.

Cymbalta is not approved for use in pediatric patients

A small number of children, teenagers, and young adults (up to 24 years of age) who took antidepressants ('mood elevators') such as duloxetine during clinical studies became suicidal (thinking about harming or killing oneself or planning or trying to do so).

Children, teenagers, and young adults who take antidepressants to treat depression or other mental illnesses may be more likely to become suicidal than children, teenagers, and young adults who do not take antidepressants to treat these conditions.

You should know that your mental health may change in unexpected ways when you take duloxetine or other antidepressants even if you are an adult over 24 years of age.

These changes may occur even if you do not have a mental illness and you are taking duloxetine to treat a different type of condition.

You may become suicidal taking this drug.

You, your family, or caregiver should call your doctor right away if you experience any of the following symptoms:

Acting without thinking
Aggressive behavior
Agitation (suddenly violent and forceful, emotionally disturbed state of mind)
Behavior changes (any other unusual changes in behavior)
Difficulty falling asleep
Difficulty staying asleep
Extreme worry
Frenzied, abnormal excitement
Hostile behavior
Irritability
New or worsening depression
Panic attacks
Planning or trying to kill yourself
Severe restlessness
Thinking about harming yourself

Thinking about killing yourself

Be sure that your family or caregiver checks on you daily so they can call the doctor if you are unable to seek treatment on your own.

Trazodone may cause painful, long lasting erections in males. In some cases emergency and/or surgical treatment has been required and, in some of these cases, permanent damage has occurred

Generic Name: triazolam
Brand Name: Halcion

Type or Class of Drug: Benzodiazepine - sedative
(One of the types of drugs used as tranquilizers or sedatives or hypnotics or muscle relaxants; chronic use can lead to dependency)

Approved for: Used to treat insomnia on a short-term basis

Dependancy and Addiction: There can be severe 'withdrawal' effects when a benzodiazepine sleeping pill is stopped.

Withdrawals: Such effects can occur after discontinuing these drugs following use for only a week or two, but may be more common and more severe after longer periods of continuous use.

Withdrawals may include:

Abdominal cramps
Convulsions (rarely)
Dysphoria (a state of anxiety, depression, unease)
Increased signs of daytime anxiety or nervousness
Mild unpleasant feelings
Muscle cramps
Perceptual disturbances
Rebound insomnia (insomnia worse than it was before)
Sweating
Tremors
Vomiting

Important Warnings:

You will probably become very sleepy soon after you take triazolam and will remain sleepy for some time after you take the medication. Plan to go to bed right after you take triazolam and to stay in bed for 7 to 8 hours. Do not take triazolam if you will be unable to remain asleep for 7 to 8 hours after taking the medication.

If you get up too soon after taking triazolam, you may experience memory problems.

Tell your doctor right away if you experience any of the following symptoms:
Aggressiveness
Confusion
Difficulty concentrating
Feeling like you are outside of your body
Hallucinations (seeing things or hearing voices that do not exist)
Memory problems
New depression
Slowed movements
Slowed speech
Strange or unusually outgoing behavior
Suicidal thoughts (thinking about killing yourself)
Worsening depression

Any other changes in your thoughts, mood or behavior.

Be sure that your family knows about these symptoms so that they can call the doctor if you are unable to seek treatment on your own.

An increase in daytime anxiety has been reported for Halcion after as few as 10 days of continuous use.

Generic Name: venlafaxine
Brand Name: Effexor / Effexor XR

Type or Class of Drug: Antidepressant

Approved for: Depression, anxiety, panic, hot flashes

Dependancy and Addiction: Your doctor will probably decrease your dose gradually. If you suddenly stop taking venlafaxine, you may experience withdrawal symptoms. Tell your doctor if you experience any of the following no matter whether you are tapering off Effexor or not.

Withdrawals: Withdrawal symptoms include:

Abnormal excitement
Agitation (suddenly violent and forceful, emotionally disturbed state of mind)
Anorexia (loss of appetite especially as result of disease)
Anxiety
Burning like feelings in any part of the body
Confusion
Diarrhea
Dizziness
Dry mouth
Electric shock like feelings in any part of the body
Fatigue
Frenzied excitement
Irritability
Lack of coordination
Loss of appetite
Nausea
Nightmares
Numbness in any part of the body
Ringing in the ears
Sad mood
Seizures
Sweating
Tingling in any part of the body
Tinnitus
Trouble falling asleep

Trouble staying asleep
Vertigo
Vomiting

Important Warnings: Effexor and Effexor XR have many warnings including the FDA's Black Box Warning. These warnings include:

Any psychoactive drug including Effexor may impair judgment, thinking, or motor skills

Antidepressants increased the risk of suicidal thinking and behavior (suicidality) in children, adolescents, and young adults.

Your mental health may change in unexpected ways when you take Effexor (venlafaxine) or other antidepressants even if you are an adult over 24 years of age.

You may become suicidal on this medication.

Patients, their families, and their caregivers should be encouraged to be alert to the emergence of the following symptoms in patients taking Effexor or Effexor XR:

Aggressiveness
Agitation (suddenly violent and forceful, emotionally disturbed state of mind)
Akathisia (A state of restlessness ranging from a feeling of inner distress to an inability to sit still)
Anxiety
Hostility
Hypomania (persistent and pervasive elated or irritable mood, and thoughts and behaviors)
Impulsivity
Insomnia
Irritability
Other unusual changes in behavior
Panic attacks
Suicidal ideation
Worsening of depression

Families and caregivers of patients should be advised to look for the emergence of such symptoms on a day-to-day basis, since changes may be abrupt.

Generic Name: zaleplon
Brand Name: Sonata

Type or Class of Drug: Hypnotic

Approved for: Used to treat insomnia (difficulty falling asleep

Dependency and Addiction: Do not stop taking Sonata without first talking to your doctor.

Withdrawals: If you suddenly stop taking zaleplon, you may experience withdrawal symptoms such as:

Muscle cramps
Seizures
Shakiness
Stomach cramps
Sweating
Unpleasant feelings
Vomiting

Important Warnings:

You should know that your mental health may change in unexpected ways while you are taking this medication.

Tell your doctor right away if you experience any of the following symptoms:

Aggressiveness
Any other changes in your usual thoughts or behavior
Confusion
Feeling as if you are outside of your body

Hallucinations (seeing things or hearing voices that do not exist)
Memory problems
New depression
Strange or unusually outgoing behavior
Thinking about killing yourself
Worsening depression

Be sure that your family knows these symptoms so that they can call the doctor if you are unable to seek treatment on your own.

Generic Name: zolpidem
Brand Name: Ambien

Type or Class: Sedative - hypnotic

Approved for: Treatment of insomnia

Dependency and Addiction: "If you take zolpidem for 2 weeks or longer, zolpidem may not help you sleep as well as it did when you first began to take the medication. If you take zolpidem for a long time, you also may develop dependence ('addiction,' a need to continue taking the medication) on zolpidem." From MedlinePlus web site

Signs of addiction include impaired control over drug use, compulsive drug use, continued use despite harm and craving.

Withdrawals: If you suddenly stop taking zolpidem, you may develop unpleasant feelings or you may experience more severe withdrawal symptoms such as:

Abdominal cramps
Convulsions
Dysphoria (a state of anxiety, depression, unease)
Fatigue
Flushing
Insomnia
Lightheadedness
Muscle cramps

Nausea
Nervousness
Panic attacks
Seizures
Shakiness
Stomach
Sweating
Tremors
Uncontrolled crying
Vomiting.

Important Warnings:

Ambien (zolpidem) may make you drowsy during the day and may increase the risk that you could fall.

Take care not to drive a car or operate machinery until you know how Ambien affects you.

Alcohol can make the side affects from Ambien worse.

Some people who took zolpidem got out of bed and drove their cars, prepared and ate food, had sex, made phone calls, or were involved in other activities while partially asleep. After they woke up, these people were usually unable to remember what they had done. Call your doctor right away if you find out that you have been driving or doing anything else unusual while you were sleeping.

Your mental health may change in unexpected ways while you are taking this medication. Notify your doctor right away if experience any of the following serious symptoms. :

Aggressiveness
Confusion
Difficulty concentrating
Extroversion that seems out of character
Hallucinations (seeing things or hearing voices that do not exist)
Feeling as if you are outside of your body
Memory problems

New or worsening depression
Slowed speech or movements
Strange or unusually outgoing behavior
Suicidal behavior
Thinking about killing yourself
Any other changes in your usual thoughts
Any other changes in your usual mood
Any other changes in your usual behavior

Be sure that your family knows these symptoms so that they can call the doctor if you are unable to seek treatment on your own.

Safety and effectiveness of Ambien have not been established in children. Many children (7.4%) given Ambien in clinical trials hallucinated (saw or heard things that were not there).

Patient Rights and Informed Consent

Patient's Rights, Patient's Freedoms and a Patient's Right to Informed Consent were all developed to protect the right of a patient within the healthcare environment. All three of these are written out here. However, the most important and the one that is legally binding is Informed Consent.

What is the Patient's Bill of Rights?

Here you will find a summary of the Consumer Bill of Rights and Responsibilities that was adopted by the *US Advisory Commission on Consumer Protection and Quality in the Health Care Industry* in 1998. It's also known as the Patient's Bill of Rights.

The Patient's Bill of Rights was created to try to reach 3 major goals:

1. To help patients feel more confident in the US health care system; the Bill of Rights:

• Assures that the health care system is fair and it works to meet patients' needs

• Gives patients a way to address any problems they may have

• Encourages patients to take an active role in staying or getting healthy

2. To stress the importance of a strong relationship between patients and their health care providers

3. To stress the key role patients play in staying healthy by laying out rights and responsibilities for all patients and health care providers

This Bill of Rights also applies to the insurance plans offered to federal employees. Many other health insurance plans and facilities have also adopted these values. Even Medicare and Medicaid stand by many of them.

The 8 key areas of the Patient's Bill of Rights

Information for patients

You have the right to accurate and easily understood information about your health plan, health care professionals, and health care facilities. If you speak another language, have a physical or mental disability, or just don't understand something, help should be given so you can make informed health care decisions.

Choice of providers and plans

You have the right to choose health care providers who can give you high-quality health care when you need it.

Access to emergency services

If you have severe pain, an injury, or sudden illness that makes you believe that your health is in danger, you have the right to be screened and stabilized using emergency services. You should be able to use these services whenever and wherever you need them, without needing to wait for authorization and without any financial penalty.

Taking part in treatment decisions

You have the right to know your treatment options and take part in decisions about your care. Parents, guardians, family members, or others that you choose can speak for you if you cannot make your own decisions.

Respect and non-discrimination

You have a right to considerate, respectful care from your doctors, health plan representatives, and other health care providers that does not discriminate against you.

Confidentiality (privacy) of health information

You have the right to talk privately with health care providers and to have your health care information protected. You also have the right to read and copy your own medical records. You have the right to ask that your doctor change your record if it is not correct, relevant, or complete.

Complaints and appeals

You have the right to a fair, fast, and objective review of any complaint you have against your health plan, doctors, hospitals or other health care personnel. This includes complaints about waiting times, operating hours, the actions of health care personnel, and the adequacy of health care facilities.

Consumer responsibilities

In a health care system that protects consumer or patients' rights, patients should expect to take on some responsibilities to get well and/or stay well (for instance, exercising and not using tobacco). Patients are expected to do things like treat health care workers and other patients with respect, try to pay their medical bills, and follow the rules and benefits of their health plan coverage. Having patients involved in their care increases the chance of the best possible outcomes and helps support a high quality, cost-conscious health care system.

Patients Freedoms

The *Association of American Physicians and Surgeons* adopted a list of patient freedoms in 1990, which was modified and adopted as a 'patients' bill of rights' in 1995:

All patients should be guaranteed the following freedoms:

To seek consultation with the physician(s) of their choice;

To contract with their physician(s) on mutually agreeable terms;

To be treated confidentially, with access to their records limited to those involved in their care or designated by the patient;

To use their own resources to purchase the care of their choice;

To refuse medical treatment even if it is recommended by their physician(s);

To be informed about their medical condition, the risks and benefits of treatment and appropriate alternatives;

To refuse third-party interference in their medical care, and to be confident that their actions in seeking or declining medical care will not result in third-party-imposed penalties for patients or physicians;

To receive full disclosure of their insurance plan in plain language

A Patient's Right to Informed Consent

Too many patients get handed a prescription by their doctor without first being given enough information to decide for themselves whether or not they should take it. You may not know this, but your doctor has a legal as well as an ethical obligation to explain to you your diagnosis as well as the benefits and potential risks associated with any medication he or she is prescribing.

In the current healthcare landscape, practitioners are under significant financial pressure to keep the time they spend with patients at a minimum. In the United States, the average doctor's appointment lasts less than 15 minutes. In the United Kingdom appointments are even shorter. This is barely enough time to find out what is bothering the person and do a minimal physical examination.

This limited time, however, is no excuse for dashing off a prescription without meeting the Informed Consent requirement.

We as patients, need to assume responsibility for our care by demanding our right to Informed Consent. If this means the appointment runs over its allotted time, so be it. Maybe the healthcare system will need to change to better allow for a real doctor-patient relationship and the true caring that implies.

What's Informed Consent?

The actual laws vary from state to state, but the bottom line is that a physician practicing in the United States must explain a diagnosis, as well as alternatives and potential risks of treatment to the patient or become potentially liable for negligence or even battery, depending on the circumstances. (Similar laws are in place in many other countries as well including Canada, Great Britain and Australia.)

Informed Consent regulations demand the information passed on to the patient be given in a way they understand. Naturally, this means the healthcare provider or a translator must communicate in a language the patient understands. That's obvious. But, how about relaying the data in terms understandable to those of us who don't have a medical degree? Too much information about potential risks can be hidden in incomprehensible (to the patient) medical terminology.

Here are the rules for Informed Consent:

The physician (not a delegated representative) should disclose and discuss:

The diagnosis, if known

The nature and purpose of a proposed treatment or procedure

The risks and benefits of proposed treatment or procedures

Alternatives (regardless of costs or extent covered by insurance)

The risks and benefits of alternatives

The risks and benefits of not receiving treatments or undergoing procedures

The most important goal of informed consent is for the patient to have the opportunity to be an informed participant in his or her own care.

The informed consent process is an opportunity for patient and physician to work together in a cooperative effort to get the best care for *you*, the patient.

Final Notes

Drug brand names are registered trademarks owned by the drug's manufacturer.
Every effort has been made to ensure that the information provided is accurate, up-to-date, and complete, but no guarantee is made to that effect. This booklet is not a substitute for medical advice or drug labeling.

The information in this booklet is in no way intended as medical advice. If you have a medical problem see a medical professional. If you are taking any pharmaceutical drug do not stop taking it without talking to a doctor.

This booklet does not include side effects and other warnings. These can be found on the labeling that came with the drug or on the FDA Medline Plus web site located here: http://www.nlm.nih.gov/medlineplus/druginformation.html. These are also available in other compilations by this writer (listed below).

One of the most important ways you can help yourself if you are taking any medication is to make sure that not only are *you* well acquainted with the potential effects of the drug but at least one *close friend or family member* is aware of those effects as well. This is especially true of pain relievers and psychoactive drugs such as antidepressants and anti-anxiety medications and antipsychotics as these can create changes in your behavior and personality of which you may not be aware.

###

Resources for Patients Rights and Informed Consent:

Patient's Bill of Rights
Patient's Freedoms
Informed Consent
HealthsourceGlobal Website (search Informed Consent)
TheFreeDictional .com (search in the legal dictionary)
www.aapsonline.org/patients/billrts.htm

References and Resources for Rest of the Book

dailymed.nlm.nih.gov/dailymed/about.cfm
www.nlm.nih.gov/medlineplus/medlineplus.html

Also available from this writer:

How Well Do You Know Your Medication?
Prescription Drug Overdose Signs and Symptoms

Antidepressants:
What Every Patient Needs to Know

Insomnia Drugs:
Side Effects and Warnings

Eat, Drink, and Be Rested
The Secret Power of Food and Natural Remedies to Help You Sleep

About the Author

Meridith Berk is a researcher and writer living in Los Angeles, CA. She writes primarily on the subject of prescription drug problems and natural solutions.

You can connect with her online at:

Twitter:
meriditht

Facebook Pages:
Natural Web MD
Eat, Drink, and be Rested
Get Off Meds
The Educated Patient Series
Prescription Drug Problems

Websites:
PrescriptionDrugProblems.com
GetOffMeds.com
TheEducatedPatientSeries.com
NaturalWebMD.com

If you like this book and find it useful, please leave a positive review. It helps.

www.ingramcontent.com/pod-product-compliance
Lightning Source LLC
Chambersburg PA
CBHW071348280526
45787CB00001B/256